mj gustner 10/98

# Memorix

The *Memorix* series consists of easy to use pocket books in a number of different medical and surgical specialities. They contain a vast amount of practical information in very concise form through the extensive use of tables and charts, lists and hundreds of clear line diagrams, often in two colours.

*Memorix* will give students, junior doctors and some of their senior colleagues a handy and comprehensive reference in their pockets.

Titles in the series include:

## Obstetrics
Thomas Rabe

## Gynecology
Thomas Rabe

## Emergency Medicine
Sönke Müller

## Neurology
Peter Berlit

## Clinical Medicine
Conrad Droste and Martin von Planta

## Surgery
Jürgen Hussmann and Robert Russell

## Physiology
Robert Schmidt, W.D. Willis and L. Reuss

## Pediatrics
Dieter Harms and Jochem Scharf

# Memorix

## Surgery

Jürgen Hussmann and
Robert C Russell

Translated by Albert Davis MD

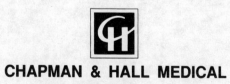

**CHAPMAN & HALL MEDICAL**
London · Weinheim · New York
Tokyo · Madras

**Published by Chapman & Hall, 2–6 Boundary Row, London SE1 8HN, UK**

Chapman & Hall, 2–6 Boundary Row, London SE1 8HN, UK

Chapman & Hall GmbH, Pappelallee 3, 69469 Weinheim, Germany

Chapman & Hall USA, 115 Fifth Avenue, New York, NY 10003, USA

Chapman & Hall Japan, ITP-Japan, Kyowa Building, 3F, 2-2-1 Hirakawacho, Chiyodaku, Tokyo 102, Japan

Chapman & Hall India, R. Seshadri, 32 Second Main Road, CIT East, Madras 600 035, India

English language edition 1997

© 1997 Chapman & Hall

Original German language edition – Memorix Spezial: Surgery © 1993, VCH Verlagsgesellschaft mbH, D-6940 Weinheim, Germany

Typeset in Times by Best-set Typesetter Ltd., Hong Kong
Printed and bound in Hong Kong

ISBN 0 412 62910 0

Apart from any fair dealing for the purposes of research or private study, or criticism or review, as permitted under the UK Copyright Designs and Patents Act, 1988, this publication may not be reproduced, stored, or transmitted, in any form or by any means, without the prior permission in writing of the publishers, or in the case of reprographic reproduction only in accordance with the terms of the licences issued by the Copyright Licensing Agency in the UK, or in accordance with the terms of licences issued by the appropriate Reproduction Rights Organization outside the UK. Enquiries concerning reproduction outside the terms stated here should be sent to the publishers at the London address printed on this page.
 The publisher makes no representation, express or implied, with regard to the accuracy of the information contained in this book and cannot accept any legal responsibility or liability for any errors or omissions that may be made.

A catalogue record for this book is available from the British Library

Library of Congress Catalog Card Number: 96-86266

# CONTENTS

| | |
|---|---|
| **Preface** | **xiii** |
| **Foreword** | **xiv** |
| **Contributors** | **xv** |

## General techniques — 1

| | |
|---|---|
| History-taking | 1 |
| Standard angles of tilt and rotation: cervical vertebrae and vertebral column | 2 |
| Standard angles of rotation: lower arm and hand | 3 |
| Standard angles of movement: shoulder and elbow | 4 |
| Standard angles of movement: vertebral column | 5 |
| Standard angles of movement: hips, knees and feet | 6 |
| Circumference and length measurements | 8 |
| Intra-articular access and injection | 9 |
| Joint punctures: shoulder, elbow and wrist | 10 |
| Joint punctures: knee and hip | 11 |
| Suture materials | 13 |
| Suturing techniques | 14 |
| Clamp–suturing techniques | 16 |

## Laboratory diagnosis — 17

| | |
|---|---|
| Hematologic values | 17 |
| Anemia | 18 |
| Evaluation of coagulation disorders | 19 |
| Coagulation disorders | 20 |
| Medications and their antidotes | 20 |
| Urinalysis | 21 |
| Differential diagnosis of surgical/urologic hematuria | 21 |

## Radiological diagnosis — 22

| | |
|---|---|
| Routine X-ray diagnosis | 22 |
| Thorax | 25 |
| Skull: lateral view | 26 |
| Skull: lateral view; common sources of error | 27 |
| Skull: occipitofrontal view | 28 |
| Skull: occipitofrontal view; common sources of error | 29 |
| Typical esophageal appearances | 30 |
| Abdominal survey | 30 |
| Joint spaces: arthritis | 31 |

# CONTENTS

| | |
|---|---|
| Normal bone development | 32 |
| Bones of the wrist | 35 |
| Bones of the foot | 36 |
| Preparation for specific radiological examinations | 37 |
| Radiological tissue densities: Hounsfield units (HU) | 38 |
| Magnetic Resonance Imaging | 39 |

## Ultrasound 42

| | |
|---|---|
| Fundamentals and indications | 42 |
| Ultrasound of internal organs | 43 |
| Ultrasound of joints and soft tissues | 45 |

## Emergencies and anesthesia 46

| | |
|---|---|
| Shock | 46 |
| Positioning | 47 |
| Resuscitation | 48 |
| Trauma: assessment and management | 50 |
| Trauma: priorities in multiple injury | 52 |
| Tracheostomy | 53 |
| Gastrointestinal (GI) bleeding | 54 |
| Upper gastrointestinal bleeding | 55 |
| Esophageal varices bleeding | 56 |
| Child classification of liver function | 56 |
| Clinical stages of hepatic encephalography | 56 |
| Thermal and chemical burns | 57 |
| Electrical injury | 60 |
| Chemical injury | 60 |
| Cold injury (hypothermia/frostbite) | 60 |
| Emergency pediatric surgery | 61 |
| Anesthesia: preparation | 66 |
| Intraoperative monitoring | 67 |
| Volume replacement | 68 |
| Intraoperative blood loss | 68 |

## Minimally invasive surgery (MIS) – special techniques 69

| | |
|---|---|
| Endoscopic surgery: fundamentals | 69 |
| Endoscopic surgery: techniques | 70 |

# CONTENTS

## Skin and soft tissue surgery and infections — 71

- Langer's skin lines — 71
- Common incisions — 72
- Local flaps — 74
- Mathes–Nahai classification of muscular blood supply — 76
- TNM classification of skin carcinoma — 77
- Differential diagnosis of melanoma — 78
- Classification of soft tissue tumors — 79
- Treatment of soft tissue tumors — 81
- Classification of soft tissue sarcomas — 82
- Wounds and wound healing — 83
- Clinical signs of acute inflammation — 84
- Disorders of wound healing — 84
- Tetanus — 85
- Gas-forming wound infections: differential diagnosis — 86
- Decubitus ulcers — 87
- Postoperative fever: differential diagnosis — 88
- Fever of undetermined origin — 89
- HIV infection/AIDS — 90

## Surgery of the face and neck — 92

- Facial fractures — 92
- Lymphoma in neck region — 93
- Lymphoma in throat region — 94
- Lateral and median throat tumors — 95

## Heart and thorax surgery — 96

- ECG/LOWN classification — 96
- Congenital heart defects — 97
- Congenital deformities of the great vessels — 100
- Acquired heart defects — 101
- Coronary arteries — 101
- Coronary surgery — 102
- Myocardial aneurysm — 103
- Acquired heart valve defects — 104
- Artificial heart valves — 105
- Heart pacemaker — 107
- New York Heart Association (NYHA) classification — 109
- Heart transplantation — 110
- Cardiac tumors — 112
- Heart–lung machine: extracorporeal circulation — 113

vii

## CONTENTS

| | |
|---|---:|
| Cardiac trauma | 114 |
| Pericardial effusion/pericardiocentesis | 115 |
| Preoperative assessment of lung function | 116 |
| Bronchial tree: lobes, segments and lymph nodes | 117 |
| Bronchoscopic views | 118 |
| Lung lobes and segments | 119 |
| Tumor diagnosis and staging | 120 |
| Histologic classification of lung tumors (WHO, 1981) | 121 |
| TNM classification of bronchial carcinoma | 122 |
| Lung surgery procedures | 123 |
| Thoracic drainage | 124 |
| Classification of mediastinal tumors | 125 |
| Mediastinal tumors: differential diagnosis | 126 |
| Pleural effusion: differential diagnosis | 127 |
| Hemoptysis/hematemesis: diagnosis | 128 |
| Chest pain: differential diagnosis | 129 |
| Chest injuries | 130 |
| Pulmonary embolus | 131 |

### Breast surgery 133

| | |
|---|---:|
| Breast tumors, mastopathy and abscesses | 133 |
| Breast cancer | 134 |

### Visceral surgery 135

| | |
|---|---:|
| Esophagus: differential diagnosis of dysphagia | 135 |
| Esophagus: atresia | 136 |
| Esophagitis and diaphragmatic hernia | 137 |
| Esophageal tumors | 138 |
| Diaphragmatic foramina: common sites of defects | 139 |
| Pelvic floor with localization of possible sites of hernia | 139 |
| Hernia | 140 |
| Diagrammatic anatomy of the inguinal region | 141 |
| Localization and relative incidence of internal hernias | 141 |
| Acute abdomen | 142 |
| Peritonitis | 145 |
| Ileus | 146 |
| Ileus: frequency related to age and cause | 147 |
| Elective ulcer surgery | 148 |
| Duodenal ulcer | 149 |
| Acute hemorrhage/perforated ulcer | 150 |
| Classification of gastric carcinoma | 151 |
| Stomach: vessels and lymph nodes | 152 |

# CONTENTS

| | |
|---|---|
| Surgery for gastric carcinoma: common procedures | 153 |
| The operated stomach | 154 |
| Small intestine: absorption and malabsorption | 155 |
| Small intestine procedures | 156 |
| TNM classification of colorectal carcinoma | 157 |
| Standard colorectal procedures | 158 |
| Artificial anus | 159 |
| Gallstones | 161 |
| Carcinoma of the biliary system | 162 |
| Liver: anatomy | 163 |
| Liver: standard resections | 164 |
| Histologic classification of liver tumors | 165 |
| Jaundice | 166 |
| Portal hypertension | 167 |
| Portal system shunt operations | 168 |
| Pancreas and pancreatitis | 169 |
| Pancreatic tumors | 170 |
| Pancreas: standard operations | 171 |
| Diverticulosis and diverticulitis of the colon | 172 |
| Crohn's disease and ulcerative colitis | 173 |
| Spleen | 174 |
| Abdominal arteries | 175 |
| Visceral arterial block | 176 |
| The retroperitoneum | 177 |
| Proctology: anal abscesses and fistulae | 178 |
| Hemorrhoids | 179 |

## Orthopedic surgery — 180

| | |
|---|---|
| Fractures | 180 |
| Fracture healing | 181 |
| Duration of healing of different bone fractures | 182 |
| Immobilization in childhood | 183 |
| AO classification of fractures: diagnostic coding | 184 |
| AO classification of fractures: humerus | 185 |
| AO classification of fractures: radius and ulna | 186 |
| AO classification of fractures: femur | 187 |
| AO classification of fractures: tibia and fibula | 188 |
| Epiphyseal fractures and growth | 189 |
| Open fractures and soft tissue damage | 190 |
| Conservative treatment of fractures | 191 |
| Bone fixation methods | 192 |
| Fracture of radius | 193 |
| Sympathetic reflex dystrophy | 193 |

## CONTENTS

| | |
|---|---:|
| Elbow or shoulder dislocation | 194 |
| Shoulder | 195 |
| Fractures of the pelvis, hip joint and femoral neck | 196 |
| Knee | 197 |
| Knee arthroscopy and functional anatomy | 198 |
| Fractures of the ankle and calcaneus | 199 |
| Fractures of the vertebral column | 200 |
| Spinal fractures: diagnosis/treatment | 201 |
| Fractures: postoperative care | 202 |
| Hardware removal | 203 |
| Aseptic bone necroses | 204 |
| Disorders of locomotion | 205 |
| Bone tumors | 206 |
| Compartment syndrome | 207 |
| Fascial divisions | 208 |
| Soft tissue defects and wound closure | 209 |
| Small bone defects | 210 |
| Large bone defects | 211 |
| Amputations and prosthetic care | 212 |

### Hand surgery  213

| | |
|---|---:|
| Replantation | 213 |
| Anesthesia | 214 |
| Common incisions | 214 |
| Relaxation position | 215 |
| Tendons and tendon injuries | 216 |
| Chronic diseases of the hand | 217 |
| Infections of the hand | 218 |
| Wound closure of hand defects | 219 |

### Endocrine surgery  220

| | |
|---|---:|
| Thyroid | 221 |
| Hyperparathyroidism | 222 |
| APUD system | 223 |
| Pheochromocytoma and endocrine pancreatic tumors | 224 |
| Gastrinoma | 225 |
| Paraneoplastic syndromes | 225 |

### Vascular surgery and the lymphatic system  226

| | |
|---|---:|
| Investigations | 226 |
| Classification of arterial aneurysms | 227 |
| Diagnosis and treatment of arterial aneurysms | 228 |

## CONTENTS

Cerebral ischemia — 229
Carotid stenosis — 230
Arterial obstruction — 231
Arteries of the pelvis — 232
Arteries of the leg — 233
Surgical treatment of vascular block — 234
Acute peripheral arterial block — 235
Acute peripheral arterial obstruction — 236
Vascular surgery: techniques — 237
Dialysis shunts — 238
Deep pelvic and femoral venous thrombosis — 239
Varicose veins: diagnosis and treatment — 241
Hodgkin's and non-Hodgkin's lymphoma — 244
Classification of lymphoid neoplasms — 245

### Neurosurgery — 246

The unconscious patient — 246
Glasgow coma and outcome scales — 247
Disorders of consciousness — 248
Craniocerebral trauma — 249
Clinical staging of craniocerebral trauma — 250
Cerebral arteries and collaterals — 252
Aneurysms — 253
Classification of subarachnoid hemorrhage — 254
The basal cisterns — 254
Intracerebral space-occupying lesions — 255
Hydrocephalus — 256
Segment innervation — 257
Spinal emergencies — 258
Spinal injuries and treatment — 259
Peripheral nerve lesions — 260
Peripheral nerve compression syndromes — 261
Disc prolapse — 262
Brain death criteria — 264

### Oncology — 265

Condition of the cancer patient — 265
Cancer staging: TNM system — 266
Tumor therapy — 266
Tumor markers — 268
Tumor of unknown origin — 269

# CONTENTS

## Treatment of pain — 270

General – acute pain — 270
Analgesics — 271
Treatment of chronic pain — 272

## Expert opinions and legal aspects — 275

Expert opinion — 275
Legal aspects of surgical practice — 276

## References — 278

## Index — 282

# PREFACE

## Preface

*Memorix* handbooks for various medical specialties have enjoyed tremendous success in Europe. The revision and updating of *Memorix Surgery* from the original German into English was a considerable challenge.

Thanks are due to the cooperation of Martin v. Planta, who conceived the idea of the first Memorix, the illustrator J. Kühn, Frau Osteen and Frau Nothacker of the VCH Publishing House, Professor A. Davis who undertook the translation, and Dr. P. Altman of Chapman & Hall Publishers, who made the preparation of this pocket surgery book possible. We are very grateful for their helpful preparatory work in the planning and progress of the project.

We thank our German and American co-authors from various disciplines for maintaining the original concept and for their professional cooperation.

Thanks are also due to the surgical teachers, medical and surgical colleagues, the medical students and many others who contributed valuable and stimulating help and practical reference work in the preparation of the book.

*Memorix Surgery* is not a replacement for standard surgical textbooks but it is meant to serve as a quick reference book containing the essential facts necessary to understand a problem, write a letter, do a dictation or refresh a memory. We hope you will find this book helpful in the daily practice of medicine.

*Jürgen Hussmann, M.D.*
*Robert C. Russell, M.D.*

# FOREWORD

## Foreword

The task of selecting and condensing essential facts from the entire spectrum of operative surgery for a quickly referenced handbook is a difficult undertaking.

*Memorix Surgery* is a successful compression of relevant surgical knowledge into a readily accessible format which is easily used by medical technologists, students, and residents.

The book is also ideal for practising physicians as a quick reference to review required anatomy, to assist in developing a definite diagnosis, and to advise non-surgical specialists of current surgical treatment options which are available. The book is organized by surgical specialty and provides the reader with easy access to topics in a given organization or area of interest.

The book is complemented by clear illustrations which are included in the text with many case-related variations from the normal, together with the appropriate diagnoses. Another advantage is the consideration given to the differential-diagnostic and therapeutic aspects provided in tabular form.

The reference list allows easy access to more permanent and detailed information.

*H.U. Steinau*

# Contributors

Greg Bennett MD
Southern Illinois University
School of Medicine
Pediatrics
P.O. Box 19230
Springfield, IL 62794-9230

F. Brandt MD
Neurosurgery
Knappschafts Hospital
D-4350 Recklinghausen

John Dietrich MD
Memorial Medical Center
Pathology
800 N. Rutledge St.
Springfield, IL 62702

Gary Draper MD
Memorial Medical Center
Anesthesiology
800 N. Rutledge St.
Springfield, IL 62702

P.W. Esser MD
Radiology
Maria-Hilf Hospital
D-4050 Mönchengladbach

K. Friedhoff MD
Surgery
Maria Hilf Hospital
Evangelical Hospital
D-4330 Mülheim/Ruhr

G. Germann MD
Burns & Plastic Surgery
BG-Trauma Hospital
D-6700 Ludwigshafen-Oggersheim

Donald R. Graham MD
Springfield Clinic
Infectious Disease
1025 S. 7th St.
Springfield, IL 62703

John Hall
Southern Illinois University
School of Medicine

Medical Student
P.O. Box 19230
Springfield, IL 62794-9230

Stephen R. Hazelrigg MD
Southern Illinois University
School of Medicine
Cardiothoracic Surgery
P.O. Box 19230
Springfield, IL 62794-9230

Jeff Higgs
Southern Illinois University
School of Medicine
Plastic and Reconstructive Surgery
P.O. Box 19230
Springfield, IL 62794-9230

Travis Hindmann MD
Memorial Medical Center
Pathology
800 N. Rutledge St.
Springfield, IL 62702

Jurgen Hussmann MD
Dept. of Plastic Surgery
BG-University Hospital
'Bergmannsheil'
P.O. Box 100250
D-44789 Bochum
Germany

Michael Johnson MD
Southern Illinois University
School of Medicine
Plastic and Reconstructive Surgery
P.O. Box 19230
Springfield, IL 62794-9230

D. Kaiser MD
Thoracic Surgery
Zehlendorf Hospital
W-1000 Berlin 39

Horst Konrad MD
Southern Illinois University
School of Medicine
Otolaryngology Surgery
P.O. Box 19230
Springfield, IL 62794-9230

# CONTRIBUTORS

F. Korsten MD
Vascular Surgery
Maria Hilf Hospital
D-4050 Mönchengladbach

John O. Kucan MD
Southern Illinois University
School of Medicine
Plastic and Reconstructive Surgery
Burn Center
P.O. Box 19230
Springfield, IL 62794-9230

J. Mathei MD
Anesthesiology, Pain Therapy
BG-University Hospital
'Bergmannsheil'
Silsinystrasse
D 44789 Bochum

Theodore R. LeBlang JD
Medical Jurisprudence
Medical Humanities
Southern Illinois University
School of Medicine
P.O. Box 19230
Springfield, IL 62794-9230

Edward J. Poje MD
Pathology
Memorial Medical Center
800 N. Rutledge St.
Springfield, IL 62702

Donald E. Ramsey MD
Southern Illinois University
School of Medicine
Vascular Surgery
P.O. Box 19230
Springfield, IL 62794-9230

Allan Roth PhD
Southern Illinois University
School of Medicine
Plastic and Reconstructive Surgery
P.O. Box 19230
Springfield, IL 62794-9230

Brian Russell MD
Springfield Clinic
Neurosurgery
455 W. Carpenter
Springfield, IL 62704

Robert C. Russell MD
Southern Illinois University School of Medicine
Plastic and Reconstructive Surgery
P.O. Box 19230
Springfield, IL 62794-9230

E. Shannon Stauffer MD
Southern Illinois University
School of Medicine
Orthopedic Surgery
P.O. Box 19230
Springfield, IL 62794-9230

M. Taupitz MD
Radiology
University Hospital
Benjamin Franklin
D-1000 Berlin 41

Roger B. Traycoff MD
Southern Illinois University
School of Medicine
Internal Medicine
P.O. Box 19230
Springfield, IL 62794-9230

Prof. Dr. K.I. Waag MD
Pediatric Surgery
Mannheim University Hospital
D-6800 Mannheim

H. Warnke MD
Cardiac Surgery
Charite
Humboldt University
D-1040 Berlin

D. Weber JD
Lawyer
D-4630 Bochum

Brian Wilson MD
Radiology
Doctors Hospital of Santa Ana
1901 North College Ave.
Santa Ana, CA 92706-2334

# Short contents

| | |
|---|---|
| General techniques | 1 |
| Laboratory diagnosis | 17 |
| Radiological diagnosis | 22 |
| Ultrasound | 42 |
| Emergencies and anesthesia | 46 |
| Minimally invasive surgery (MIS) – special techniques | 69 |
| Skin and soft tissue surgery and infections | 71 |
| Surgery of the face and neck | 92 |
| Heart and thorax surgery | 96 |
| Breast surgery | 133 |
| Visceral surgery | 135 |
| Orthopedic surgery | 180 |
| Hand surgery | 213 |
| Endocrine surgery | 220 |
| Vascular surgery and the lymphatic system | 226 |
| Neurosurgery | 246 |
| Oncology | 265 |
| Treatment of pain | 270 |
| Expert opinions and legal aspects | 275 |
| References | 278 |
| Index | 282 |

# GENERAL TECHNIQUES

## History-taking
### Chief complaint

**History of the present illness**
  Onset
  Duration
  Associated symptoms (e.g. weight loss, fever, loss of appetite)
**Past medical history**
  Current or previous physicians and diagnoses (e.g. hypertension, asthma, bleeding disorders, liver disease, rheumatic fever, tuberculosis, venereal disease)
  Significant childhood illnesses
  Previous hospitalizations, operations or accidents
  Previous blood transfusions
**Family history**
  Name, age, address, date of birth
  Name and address of spouse, closest kin or guardian
  Inherited familial disorders (e.g. hemophilia, von Willebrand's disease)
  Cause of death in nearest relatives
  Recent illnesses in the immediate family
**Social history**
  Marital status
  Occupation, hobbies and leisure activities
  Sexual history
  Alcohol, nicotine, coffee, illegal drugs
  Smoking history
**Medications:** (anticoagulants, antihypertenssives, antidepressants, digitalis, oral contraceptives, immunosuppressive agents, steroids)

Allergies: medications, insect bites, etc.

### Review of systems
  **Skin:** color, pigmentation, petechiae, purpura, pigmented lesions, café au lait spots, easy bruising
  **Cardiopulmonary:** dyspnea on exertion, hoarseness, cough, hematemesis, chest pain, nocturnal urinary frequency, dependent edema, headache, vertigo, palpitations, syncopal episodes
  **GI:** regurgitation, heartburn, vomiting, dysphagia, constipation, change in bowel habits or character of stools
  **Urogenital:** frequency, dysuria, dyspareunia, impotence, abnormal vaginal bleeding, edema, excessive thirst
  **Neurologic:** changes in sensation (tingling, hyperesthesia, paralysis, altered sensorium, trembling, spasm, auditory of visual changes, change in speech or behavior
  **Musculoskeletal:** cramps, pains, impaired movement, abnormal gait
  **Hematologic:** easy fatigue, dyspnea, petechiae, abnormal bleeding (purpura, nosebleeds, joint bleeding, excessive menstrual bleeding), bone pain (leukemia, multiple myeloma), lymphadenopathy

### Physical examination
  Vital signs: pulse and BP (both supine and standing if indicated), temperature
  HEENT: ears
  Chest: symmetry, expansion, dullness, rales
  Abdomen: tenderness, palpable mass
  Genitourinary
  Neurologic: cranial nerves, fundoscopic examination
  Extremities
  Skin

### Chest X-ray
### Laboratory investigations

## MEMORIX SURGERY

## Standard angles of tilt and rotation: cervical vertebrae and vertebral column

**Measuring point: foramen ovale**

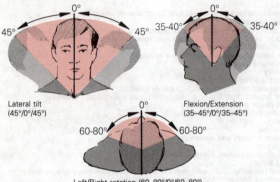

Lateral tilt
(45°/0°/45°)

Flexion/Extension
(35–45°/0°/35–45°)

Left/Right rotation (60–80°/0°/60–80°)

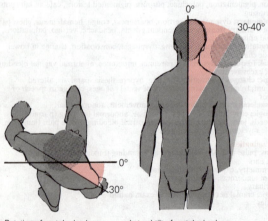

Rotation of vertebral column
(30°/0°/30°)

Lateral tilt of vertebral column
(30–40°/0°/30–40°)

## GENERAL TECHNIQUES

# Standard angles of rotation: Lower arm and hand

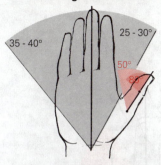

Radial abduction, ulnar abduction at hand joint (25–30°/0°/35–40°)
Flexion of thumb at MP joint (50°/0°/0°)
Flexion of thumb at IP joint (80°/0°/0°)

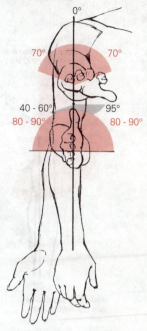

Pronation, supination of forearm (80–90°/0°/80–90°)
Medial rotation, lateral rotation (70°/0°/70°)

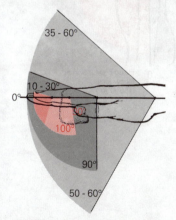

---

MP: metacarpophalangeal
IP: interphalangeal
(P: proximal; D: distal)
PIP: proximal interphalangeal
DIP: distal interphalangeal

Flexion, extension at wrist joint (50–60°/0°/35–60°)
Flexion, extension of finger at MP joint (90°/0°/10–30°)
Flexion of finger at PIP joint (100°/0°/0°)
Flexion of finger at DIP joint (90°/0°/0°)

## MEMORIX SURGERY

## Standard angles of movement: shoulder and elbow

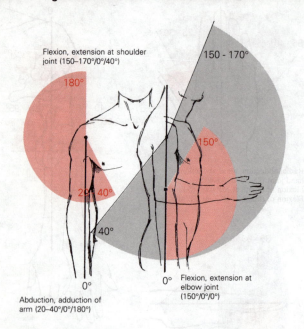

Flexion, extension at shoulder joint (150–170°/0°/40°)

Abduction, adduction of arm (20–40°/0°/180°)

Flexion, extension at elbow joint (150°/0°/0°)

## GENERAL TECHNIQUES

# Standard angles of movement: vertebral column

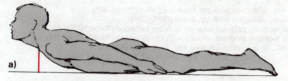

a) Finger–floor distance. Spine extension in the prone position

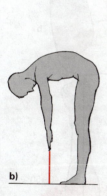

b) Finger–floor distance. Trunk flexion with extended knees

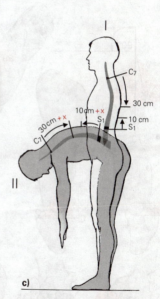

c)

### Schober's sign

I  Mark a skin point 30 cm caudal to $C_7$, and a second 10 cm cranial to $S_1$ in the erect position
II Measure distally from $C_7$ to the skin point (30 cm + x cm). Also measure from $S_1$ proximally to the skin point (10 cm + x cm), each time after active flexion with the knees extended

## MEMORIX SURGERY

## Standard angles of movement: hips, knees and feet

a Abduction, adduction with hip extended (30–45°/0°/20–30°)
b Abduction, adduction with hip flexed (80°/0°/20°)
  Internal rotation, external rotation with hip extended (40–50°/0°/30–45°)
c Internal rotation, external rotation with hip extended (30–40°/0°/40–50°)
d Pronation, supination of forefoot with fixed heel (15°/0°/35°)
e Eversion, inversion in subtalar joint (30°/0°/60°)

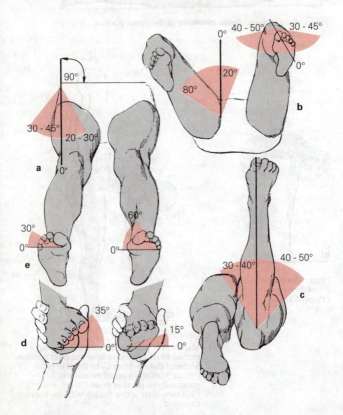

## GENERAL TECHNIQUES

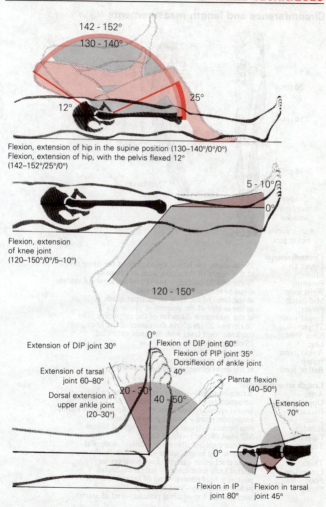

Flexion, extension of hip in the supine position (130–140°/0°/0°)
Flexion, extension of hip, with the pelvis flexed 12° (142–152°/25°/0°)

Flexion, extension of knee joint (120–150°/0°/5–10°)

Extension of DIP joint 30°
Flexion of DIP joint 60°
Flexion of PIP joint 35°
Dorsiflexion of ankle joint 40°
Extension of tarsal joint 60–80°
Plantar flexion (40–50°)
Dorsal extension in upper ankle joint (20–30°)
Extension 70°
Flexion in IP joint 80°
Flexion in tarsal joint 45°

## Circumference and length measurements

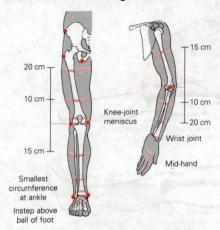

**Circumferences:**
| | |
|---|---|
| Upper arm: | 15 cm above the lateral epicondyle of the humerus |
| Elbow: | at the height of the elbow joint in extension |
| Forearm: | 10 cm and 20 cm below the lateral humeral epicondyle |
| Wrist joint: | distal to the radius and ulna styloid |
| Mid-hand: | at the level of the II–V metacarpal heads |
| Finger: | in the center of the respective phalanges |
| Finger joint: | at the maximum diameter of the respective joint |
| Thigh: | 10 cm and 20 cm above the center of the knee joint |
| Knee joint: | the knee joint level with the knee extended |
| Leg: | 15 cm below the mid-knee joint |
| Ankle joint: | above the malleoli |
| Instep: | above the navicular bone |
| Ball of foot: | at the level of metatarsal heads I–V |

**Length measurements:**
| | |
|---|---|
| Arm: | acromion point – styloid process of the radius |
| Upper arm: | acromion point – lateral epicondyle of the humerus |
| Forearm: | lateral epicondyle of humerus – styloid process radius |
| Ulna: | olecranon point – styloid process of ulna |
| Hand: | line between styloid processes – tips of fingers |
| Finger: | MP joint (flexed) – tip of finger |
| True leg: | anterior superior iliac spine – lateral malleolus<br>apparent leg length, navel – medial malleolus |
| Thigh: | great trochanter – lateral knee joint center |
| Lower leg: | lateral knee joint center – lateral malleolus |
| Foot: | posterior heel border – end of longest toe |
| Stump: | ischial tuberosity – end of stump<br>lateral knee, top of tibial plateau – end of stump |

## GENERAL TECHNIQUES

# Intra-articular access and injection

**Essential preparation**
- Careful diagnostic assessment
- Explanation of the procedure and risks, and alternative methods

**Contraindications**
- Skin infection or skin disease in the vicinity of the injection site. (In penetrating puncture, the needle should be placed as far away from the affected area as possible.)

**Room requirements**
- Equipment in accordance with the sterile requirements of the operation room
- With contamination by bacteria or with uncertainty about the sterility of the room, the operation is best carried out with single-use instruments and water-resistant drapes
- During the operative preliminaries excessive movement and talking among the personnel should be at a minimum to restrict possible infection
- Use of face mask and sterile gloves

**Preparation of the patient**
- Adequate exposure (remove clothes from the operative field)
- Shave area
- Wash area
- Sterilization of the injection site and surrounding area, after previous cleaning (avoid skin damage from shaving)
- Apply disinfectant
- Leave adequate time for the disinfectant to work

**Surgeon, personnel**
- To prevent contamination roll up sleeves to above elbows
- Meticulous hand scrub
- Use sterile gloves for the entire procedure, including syringe handling

**Injection preparations**
- Use single-use syringes and needles
- Open sterile packs immediately before use

**Postoperatively**
- Dress the puncture area with a gauze bandage

**Final care**
- For severe pain in the operative area, call for specialist consultation
- Dispose of all contaminated dressings and instruments carefully and completely to avoid spread of infection

# MEMORIX SURGERY

## Joint punctures: shoulder, elbow and wrist

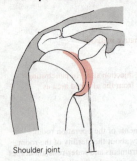
Shoulder joint

**From the front:** on the anterior border of the deltoid, 1 cm below the coracoid process
**From behind:** below the acromion in line with the coracoid process

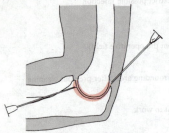
Elbow joint

**From behind:** with 90° elbow flexion, directly above the olecranon
**From the side:** with 90° elbow flexion, between the lateral humeral epicondyle and the head of the radius

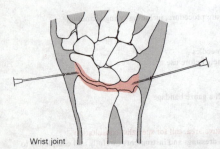
Wrist joint

**From radial side:** distal to the radial styloid process and radial to the tendon of the extensor pollicis longus
**From ulnar side:** volar to the tendon of the extensor minimi
**From dorsal side:** radially to the tendon of the extensor indicis

## GENERAL TECHNIQUES

## Joint punctures: knee and hip

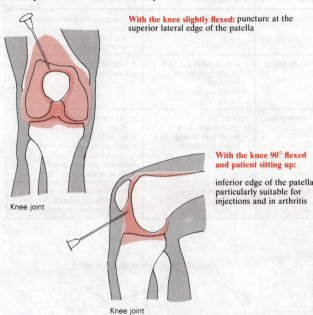

**With the knee slightly flexed:** puncture at the superior lateral edge of the patella

Knee joint

**With the knee 90° flexed and patient sitting up:**

inferior edge of the patella particularly suitable for injections and in arthritis

Knee joint

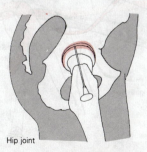

**From the side:** with the patient lying on the opposite side, above the trochanter

Hip joint

## MEMORIX SURGERY

| Vein | Peripheral | Central |
|---|---|---|
| Advantages | • technically simple<br>• signs of infection appear early | • necessary for total parenteral nutrition<br>• accessible subclavian vein even with patient in shock |
| Disadvantages | • not available for high calorie parenteral nutrition<br>• venous collapse in shock | • technically more difficult and expensive |
| Complications | • infection<br>• thrombophlebitis<br>• vessel wall damage by highly concentrated solutions | • pneumothorax (hemato-, chylo-, infusion thorax)<br>• air embolism<br>• arterial puncture<br>• sepsis/infection<br>• thrombosis/hematoma<br>• thromboembolism |
| Indications | • low invasive risk<br>• rapid access needed | • total parenteral nutrition<br>• IV antibiotics/chemotherapy<br>• hemodynamic measurements |

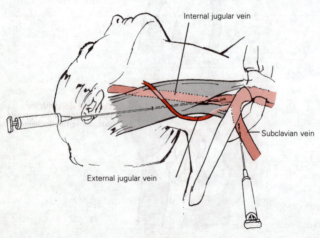

## GENERAL TECHNIQUES

## Suture materials

Traumatic: suture threaded into needle
Atraumatic: thread integrated into needle, minimal tissue trauma
Absorbable: fermentative or hydrolytic breakdown
Non-absorbable: loss of tensile strength over months or years
Monofil: homogeneous structure, minimal tissue reaction, poor knot security
Polyfil: twisted, braided, wick effect, good knot security
Pseudomonofil: polyfil with layered surface, combines advantages of the two previously described thread structures

|  | Suture material | Tissue reaction | Properties | Application |
|---|---|---|---|---|
| **Non-absorbable** | | | | |
| Metal wires<br>Metal clips<br>Metal staples | Chrome–iron–nickel combinations, monofil, polyfil | | High tensile strength; breaks with strong turn only; minimal tissue trauma | Fascia (burst abdomen), tendon, bone, skin, bronchus |
| Polypropylene | Monofil | | Minimal tissue reaction; long-lasting 3 to 4-knot flexibility | Tendons, blood vessels, skin, universal use |
| Polyamide | Monofil | | High tensile strength; minimal tissue reaction | Tendons, vessels, skin |
| Polyester | Twisted, braided | | Better flexibility and knot stability | Tendons, vessels, skin |
| Silk | Twisted, braided | | High tensile strength; very good flexibility; tissue inflammation; very good knot stability | Large vessels |
| Cotton | | | | Large vessels (rarely) |
| **Absorbable** | | | | |
| Polydioxanon | Monofil | | Minimal tissue reaction; good flexibility; high tensile strength | Tendons, fascia, muscle parenchymal tissue, gynecology |
| Polyglycolate | Monofil | | | |
| Polyglycolic acid | Braided, layered | | High tensile strength; complete absorption, good knot security | Fascia, parenchymal tissue, gynecology |
| Chromic catgut | Monofil, tanned with chromic acid | | Complete absorption; strong tissue reaction; moderate knot security; variable tensile strength | Mucosa, bladder, parenchymal tissues, muscle |

## MEMORIX SURGERY

## Suturing techniques

### Principles of surgical suturing

– Avoid further injury to the skin wound margins by gentle handling of tissue (use toothed forceps, single hooks, or stay sutures to gently approximate skin wound edges)
– All non-viable or contaminated tissue in traumatic wounds should be débrided and irrigated thoroughly before wound closure
– Sutures should be placed at equal distance and depth from the wound edge
– Approximate wound edges without tension; sutures should not strangulate tissue
– Avoid leaving cavities or dead space which can accumulate fluid
– Place knots on the better-vascularized wound edge
– If the condition of the wound is uncertain, do not attempt primary closure

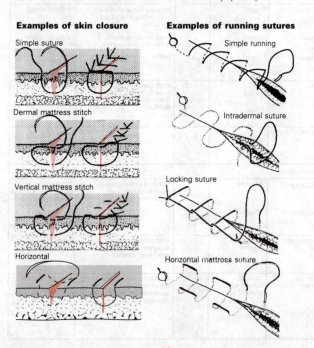

**Examples of skin closure**
- Simple suture
- Dermal mattress stitch
- Vertical mattress stitch
- Horizontal

**Examples of running sutures**
- Simple running
- Intradermal suture
- Locking suture
- Horizontal mattress suture

## GENERAL TECHNIQUES

**Examples of gastrointestinal sutures**

Single row, layered

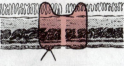

Mucosa
Submucosa
Muscularis
Serosa

*Double row*, layered, inverted

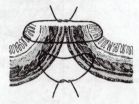

Mucosa
Submucosa
Muscularis
Serosa

**Principles for the removal of non-absorbable sutures or staples:**
– one side of the stitch should be cut at the skin level
– skin staples are removed with a staple remover
– facial suture should be removed in 3–5 days and held with skin tape if necessary to prevent permanent 'stitch marks'
– intradermal sutures can be left for 3 weeks or longer

## *MEMORIX SURGERY*

## Clamp–suturing techniques

**Example:**
**1. Application of a double-row clamp–suture**
(e.g. closure of a bronchial stump; removal of a diverticulum)

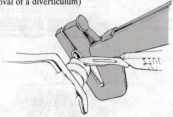

**2. Application of two double-row clamp–sutures**
(e.g. closure of lung or bowel segments; small bowel anastomosis)

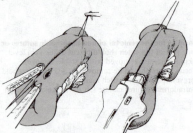

**3. Making a circular anastomosis**
(e.g. esophagojejunostomy after gastrectomy; low rectal resection)

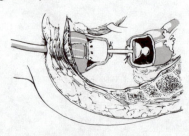

# LABORATORY DIAGNOSIS

## Hematologic values

### Normal blood count

| | | |
|---|---|---|
| Hemoglobin (g/dl) | Women | 12–16 |
| | Men | 14–18 |
| Hematocrit (%) | Women | 37–47 |
| | Men | 41–51 |
| Erythrocytes ($\times 10^6$) | Women | 4:0–5:5 |
| | Men | 4:5–6:0 |
| Median corpuscular volume (MCV) | Hematocrit ×10: erythrocytes | |
| | Normal: 85 fl | |
| Median corpuscular hemoglobin (MCH) | Hemoglobin ×10: erythrocytes | |
| | Normal: 29 pg | |
| Median corpuscular hemoglobin concentration (MCHC) | Hemoglobin ×100: hematocrit | |
| | Normal: 34 g/dl | |
| Reticulocytes | Normal: 10–20‰ | |
| Leukocytes | Normal: 4000–10 000 | |
| Thrombocytes | Normal: 150 000–400 000 | |

| Differential blood count (%) | |
|---|---|
| Polymorphonuclear neutrophils | 40–70 |
| Band neutrophils | 5–15 |
| Eosinophils | 2–10 |
| Basophils | 0–1 |
| Lymphocytes | 20–40 |
| Monocytes | 2–10 |

### Erythrocyte sedimentation rate (ESR)

Normal value (Westergren): 10 mm after 1 h
20 mm after 2 h

**Expected results** in acute and chronic infections

| ↑↑↑ | ↑↑ | ↑ | Normal | ↓ |
|---|---|---|---|---|
| Thyroiditis, polyarthritis, peritonitis, sepsis, malignancy, plasmocytoma, Hodgkin's disease, rheumatic fever, temporal arteritis, collagen diseases | Osteomyelitis, cholecystitis, pancreatitis, appendicitis, liver diseases, myocardial infarction, malignancy | Postoperative anemia, leukemia, tuberculosis | Does not exclude a pathological process | Jaundice, polycythemia, congestive heart failure |

# MEMORIX SURGERY

## Anemia

**Etiology**
Bleeding, bleeding disorders, hemolytic anemia

**Diagnosis**
History, physical examination, hemoglobin, hematocrit, erythrocytes, serum iron, ferritin, transferrin, reticulocytes, blood specimen, bone marrow puncture, thyroid function studies, cortisol, LDH, Coomb's test, folic acid, vitamin $B_{12}$, hemoglobin-electrophoresis

| Classification | | |
|---|---|---|
| Normocytic | Microcytic | Macrocytic |
| Median corpuscular volume (MCV) 85–95 $\mu m^3$ | MCV < 85 $\mu m^3$ | MCV > 95 $\mu m^3$ |
| *Acute blood loss,* chronic blood loss, inflammatory diseases, (e.g. osteomyelitis), endrocrinopathy, liver and renal diseases, neoplasms, hemolysis (infection, medicinal, toxemic, immunologic, microangiopathic), bone marrow deficiency | Iron deficiency (e.g. after gastrectomy) hemoglobinopathy, sideroblastic anemia, inflammatory diseases, neoplasms | Vitamin $B_{12}$ deficiency (e.g. in chronic, atrophic gastritis, gastrectomy), folic acid deficiency, aplastic anemia, liver diseases |
| **Treatment** | | |
| (Fresh blood) Concentrated erythrocytes, fresh frozen plasma | $FeSO_4$ by mouth (e.g. 2 × 100 mg beginning with 100 mg/day), parenterally many side effects possible, pyridoxin | Vitamin $B_{12}$ parenterally, folic acid |

## LABORATORY DIAGNOSIS

# Evaluation of coagulation disorders

### History

Example: frequent nosebleeds, hematuria, trivial local trauma bleeds, prolonged bleeding following injection, puncture, injury or tooth extraction, bleeding complications during or after past surgical procedures, menorrhagia, liver disease, renal disease

### Physical examination

Example: petechiae (small punctiform hemorrhages), purpura (generalized petechiae), ecchymoses (superficial enclosed bleeding), hematoma, microcirculation disorders

### Bleeding time (Duke)

To test for thrombocyte function and extent of the bleeding propensity, make a 3–5-mm-deep incision by lancet and aspirate blood without contacting the wound. Normal value 1–3.5 min, pathological in severe disturbance of the primary bleeding phase, thrombocytopenia, von Willebrand's disease, thrombasthenia, result of medication

### Rumpel–Leede test

Test of capillary resistance by pressure loading on the upper arm

$$\frac{systole + diastole}{2}$$

Example: with the blood pressure cuff on for 10 min; normal value 3–10 petechiae, pathological with vascular damage or severe thrombocyte damage

### Laboratory diagnosis

– To exclude all possible coagulation disorders by a screening program is senseless and impractical. Specific questioning and examination is required.

---

**Basic diagnosis**
- Thrombocyte count
- Quick-test (exogenous system)
- Activated partial thromboplastin time (aPTT) (endogenous system)
- Fibrin stabilization test

---

**Special diagnostic methods**

# MEMORIX SURGERY

## Coagulation disorders

| Medications possibly causing coagulation disorders | |
|---|---|
| Acetylsalicylic acid<br>Actinomycin D<br>Allopurinol<br>Ampicillin<br>Asparaginase<br>Bleomycin<br>Busulfan<br>Quinine<br>Chlorambucil<br>Chloramphenicol<br>Chlordiazepoxide<br>Chlorthiazide<br>Chlorpromazine<br>Chlorpropamide<br>Cimetidine<br>Colchicine<br>Cyclophosphamide<br>Cytarabine<br>Diazepam<br>Fluorouracil | Furosemide<br>Gold<br>Heparin<br>Indomethacin<br>Lidocaine<br>Lincomycin<br>Mercaptopurine<br>Metamizol<br>Methicillin<br>Methotrexate<br>Methyldopa<br>Oxyphenbutazone<br>Paracetamol<br>Phenylbutazone<br>Phenytoin<br>Streptomycin<br>Sulfonamide<br>Tolbutamide<br>Vinblastine<br>Vincristine |

## Medications and their antidotes

| Medication | Antidote |
|---|---|
| **Heparin**<br>Action: antithrombin<br>inactivates IIa, IX, X; inhibits the conversion of prothrombin to thrombin, develops its action in the presence of heparin factor (antithrombin III)<br>Short half-life | **Protamine** |
| **Coumarin**<br>Action: Vitamin K antagonist inactivates II, VII, IX, X<br>Long half-life | **Vitamin $K_1$**<br>It is used in the liver for the synthesis of factors II, VII, IX, X |
| **Fibrinolytics**<br>**Streptokinase, urokinase**<br>Action: promotes the conversion of plasminogen to plasmin | **Antifibrinolytics**<br>**Tranexaminic acid, Epsilon-aminocaproic acid**<br>Action: inhibits the activation of plasminogen |

# LABORATORY DIAGNOSIS

## Urinalysis

Screening investigation: erythrocytes/hemoglobin, albumin, glucose, ketones, nitrites, pH

**Urine sediment**

|  | Normal |
|---|---|
| Erythrocytes | ≤4 per field |
| Leukocytes | ≤6 per field |
| Bacteria | None |
| Crystals | None |
| Cylinders | None |

**Cytology**
Dysplasia, cytological malignant criteria

## Differential diagnosis of surgical/urologic hematuria

**Microhematuria:** erythrocytes in urine
**Macrohematuria:** blood in urine visible to naked eye

**Trauma:** e.g. contusion of kidney – rupture, bladder or urethral injury, insertion of suprapubic catheter

**Stones:** in renal pelvis or calyces, ureter, bladder, urethra

**Tumors:** of renal parenchyma, renal pelvis, ureter, bladder, prostate, urethra

**Infection:** glomerulonephritis, pyelonephritis, hemorrhagic cystitis

**Anticoagulant treatment**

**March hematuria:** after extreme physical effort

**Hemorrhagic diathesis**

**Internal causes:** (infarct, infectious diseases, hypertension, nephrosclerosis, toxemia, papillary necrosis, blood diseases, menstrual blood contamination)

## MEMORIX SURGERY

## Routine X-ray diagnosis
(Standard X-ray photography and the common specialized X-rays)

**Skull**
Skull p.-a. – facial bones, nasal sinuses, frontal sinuses
Skull in Altschul's projection – posterior skull, occipital bone, foramen magnum
Skull a.-p. with mouth open – teeth, upper cervical vertebrae
Skull lateral – lateral skull area, maxillary joint, base of skull
Schuller's projection – mastoid process, external auditory canal, maxillary joint
Stenvers projection – labyrinth complex, internal auditory canal
Rhese projection – optic canal
Occipitonasal – frontal sinuses
Occipitomental with mouth open – maxillary sinuses, ethmoid cells, floor of orbit

**Vertebral column**
Upper, mid-, lower spine a.-p.
Upper, mid-, lower spine laterally
Oblique pictures – intervertebral foramina, small vertebral joints
Function photographs – segment movement blocking, segmental ligament hypermobility

**Ribs**
Thorax a.-p. – posterior rib sector
Thorax oblique – anterior rib sector
Thorax tangential, target photographs – details

**Sternum**
Sternum laterally
LAO – breathing technique

**Shoulder**
Shoulder a.-p. (arms hanging) – dislocation of the acromioclavicular joint
Shoulder in glenoid-tangential projection – superimposition-free photograph of head of humerus and joint socket

Profile anomaly suggests separation of the acromio-clavicular joint

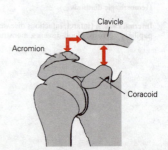

# RADIOLOGICAL DIAGNOSIS

## Routine X-ray diagnosis
Y-photographs (the acromion, coracoid and tangential scapula make the shaft of the 'Y')
– dislocation of shoulder (two level planes; see the figure on p. 22)

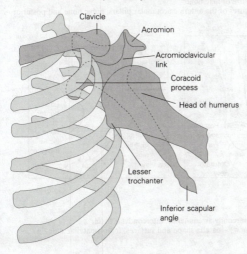

Shoulder transthoracic – subcapital fracture
Target photograph – e.g. for suspected Bankart lesion or Hill–Sachs defect

**Elbow**
Elbow a.-p.
Elbow lateral
Elbow in oblique projection – head of radius, coronoid process

**Hand**
Hand dorsopalmar
Hand lateral
Navicular group – scaphoid fracture

**Thorax**
Thorax p.-a. (see the figure on p. 25)
Thorax lateral

**Abdomen**
Abdominal general (standing and sitting)
Abdomen left-sided
Abdomen empty (lying)

# MEMORIX SURGERY

**Pelvis**
Pelvis general
Axial hip, after Lauenstein
View of the ala – fracture of iliac bone
Obturator view – fractures of the anterior acetabular pillars, pubic bone and posterior pillars

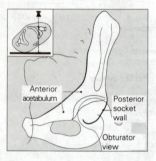
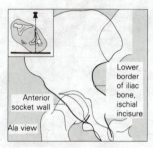

**Knee**
Knee a.-p.
Knee lateral
Frik's tunnel view – intercondylar eminence, intercondylar fossa
Patella axial (sunrise view) – patella shape and surfaces, femoropatellar slide

**Ankle**
Ankle a.-p.
Ankle lateral
Sustained views – talar angle; anterior dislocation of talus

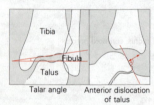

Talar angle: 7°
Anterior dislocation of talus: 7 mm
Δ Contralateral foot: 5°/5 mm

**Foot**
Foot a.-p.
Foot dorsoplantar in oblique projection
Foot plantodorsal in oblique projection (patient prone) – medial basal bones of foot (medial cuneiform, intermedial cuneiform)
Foot lateral – calcaneous
Foot axial – calcaneus

(From Häring, R. and Zilch, H. (1990))

## RADIOLOGICAL DIAGNOSIS

## Thorax

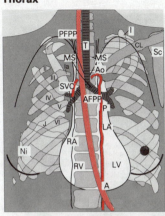

| | |
|---|---|
| I | 1st Rib |
| II | Anterior portion of 2nd rib |
| III–VI | Posterior part of 3rd–6th rib |
| Ia | Cartilage of 1st rib |
| J | Interlobar line |
| MS | Manubrium sterni |
| CL | Clavicle |
| Ni | Nipple |
| Sc | Scapula |
| T | Trachea |
| PFPP | posterior fold of parietal pleura |
| AFPP | anterior fold of parietal pleura |

*Heart*

| | |
|---|---|
| Ao | Aortic button – distal area of aortic arch |
| SVC | Superior vena cava |
| P | Pulmonary trunk |
| RA | Right atrium |
| LA | Left atrium |
| RV | Right ventricle |
| LV | Left ventricle |

## Most frequent causes of diagnostic error

(From Freye, K. and Lammers, W. (1985))

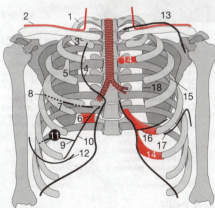

1. Cervical rib
2. Contour of sternocleidomastoid m.
3. Shadow of 1st and 2nd ribs
4. Azygos vein lobe
5. Articular bone break between 1st and 2nd rib in front
6. Firm bone break between 5th and 6th rib behind
7. Bifurcation of 3rd rib
8. Interlobar line between upper and middle lobes (minor fissure)
9. Deep-seated accessory interlobar lines of the lower lobe apex
10. Cardiac lobe
11. Nipple
12. Mammary shadow
13. Subclavian artery
14. Calcified rib cartilage
15. Costal sulcus
16. Interlobar line of an accessory left middle lobe
17. Pectoralis shadow
18. Border of scapula

## MEMORIX SURGERY

## Skull: lateral view

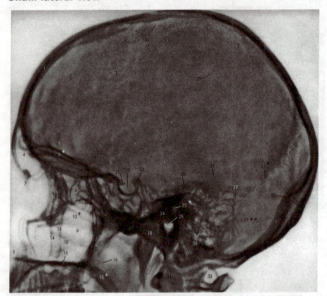

1. Frontal bone
2. Parietal bone
3. Coronal suture
4. Frontal sinus
5. Roof of posterior, anterior orbit
6. Ethmoid cells
7. Nasal bone
8. Anterior nasal spine
9. Maxillary sinus
10. Inferior, middle, nasal concha
11. Outer margin of anterior
12. and posterior orbit
13. Zygomatic process (cross-cut view) near and
14. far sides
15. Hard palate
15*. Soft palate
16. Pterygoid process
17. Condylar process
18. Head of mandible
19. Sphenoidal sinuses
20. Sella turcica
21. Anterior clinical process
22. Posterior clinical process
23. Groove for the middle meningeal artery
24. Pars petrosa area
25. External acoustic
25*. Internal acoustic
26. Foramen magnum region
27. Parietomastoid suture
27*. Lambdoid suture
27**. Occipitomastoid suture
28. Concha of ear
29. Diploic canals, extended in network
30. Arachnoid polyps (Pacchioni granules)
31. Groove for middle meningeal artery
32. Posterior wall of pharynx
33. Arcuate foramen of Atlas
34. Teeth
35. Internal occipital protuberance

(From Grashey, R. and Birkner, R. (1964))

## RADIOLOGICAL DIAGNOSIS

## Skull: lateral view; common sources of error

Cc Persistent patent craniopharyngeal canal
ct Thyroid cartilage
f Petrous bone
j Juga cerebralis
k Hyperostotic fused coronal suture
l Occasionally encountered light lines mimicking fissures. They can simulate the grooves of branches of the middle meningeal artery
m External acoustic meatus
Ps Suboccipital process
sh Stylohyoid ligament
th Thyrohyoid ligament, ossified, as continuation of the hyoid cornu

11* Transverse occipital suture only laterally formed: a false suture
14* Calcified internal carotid (possible to be mistaken for intracellular calcification)
21 Ossified dura
22 Suture
23 Overlapping suture
24 Parietozygomatic suture, branch from the lambdoid suture to the squamous suture
25 Pseudo-compression fracture, from vessel walls or other uneven lines on the internal table
26 Occipital spur, the external occipital protuberance mostly in older people becomes a spur against the nuchal ligament
27 Auricle, blocked ear requires greater projection
28 Frontozygomatic suture. This suture can gape and then be taken for a fracture
29 Hyperostosis of frontal bone
29* Middle temporal diploic vein, flows generally in the foveola granularis
30 Deep course sulcus of a branch of the meningeal artery, can be mistaken for a fracture
31 Styloid process, normal 2-3 cm, can prolong to 6-7 cm
31 Partial ossification of stylohyoid ligament with joint-like subdivision
32 Nasomaxillary suture
32* Groove for the anterior ethmoid artery and nerve
33 Mandibular canal, widened conspicuously above. The mylohyoid line lies on the inner side of the mandible, and the same muscle arises in this area. Overprojection of this sharp line on the mandibular canal can cause apparent widening
36 Cellular mastoids. Above: sigmoid sinus as continuation of the transverse sinus. Many veins, varying in number, position and width
37 Calcified 'wheat ear' cartilage. Sesamoid bones within the thyrohyoid ligament projecting between the horns of hyoid and superior thyroid cartilage
45 Spondylarthrosis deformans
46,47 Calcinosis circumscripta of ligamenta nuchae. Diff.-diag: 1. persistent apophyseal nucleus 2. fatigue fracture (spade fracture) of 7th spinous process. The fracture lies in the base of the process
48 Fissure in hyoid bone. The connection with the hyoid can be completely absent
49 Arcuate foramen. Formation of canal forte vertebral artery and suboccipital nerve on the atlas. The canal is formed by a bony clasp which runs from the posterior occipital socket of the atlas to its dorsal bend.

(From Grashey, R. and Birkner, R. (1964))

# MEMORIX SURGERY

## Skull: occipitofrontal view

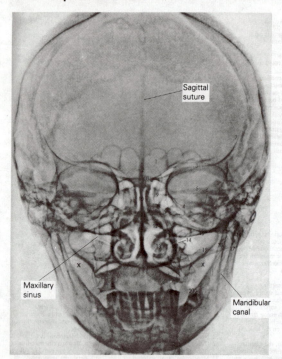

1 Frontal sinus (asymmetry is common)
2 Frontal sinus septum
3 Roof of orbit
4 Floor of orbit
5 Petrous bone
6 Cochlea
7 Part of the lateral skull wall, at the border of the anterior and middle cavities
8 Base of the anterior skull cavity
9 Ethmoidal labyrinth
10 Median septum of the lateral cavities, below: osseous nasal septum
11 Base of skull with floor of sphenoid sinus
12 Medial nasal concha
13 Inferior nasal concha
14 Atlanto-occipital joint
15 Base of posterior and middle skull cavity
16 Mastoid process
17 Condylar process
18 Coronoid process
19 Zygomatic bone
20 Retained root with periapical absorption area. Upper jaw edentulous, lower jaw with defective bite
21 Sagittal suture
22 Maxillary sinus
23 Mandibular canal

(After Grashey, R. and Birkner, R. (1964))

# RADIOLOGICAL DIAGNOSIS

## Skull: occipitofrontal view; common sources of error

1 Persistent frontal suture. Can be mistaken if the sagittal suture projects, because of deep insertion of the sagittal suture into the frontal bone. Occasionally there is a gap (metopic fontanelle) in the lower third of the frontal suture, or such gaps can be ossified (os metopicum). The fonticulus metopicus is often combined with a frontal hyperostosis. Non-union of both is also found in craniocleido dystosis
2 Ossified falx cerebri
3 Calcified pineal gland. The calcified image must be photographed from the side sagittally in the median plane. In pathological conditions the calcified gland shadow can be displaced laterally or forward. The pineal gland normally lies 4 cm above and 1 cm dorsal to the porus acousticus.
4 Crista galli. The lamina perpenducularis projects into the anterior cranial cavity
5 Frontal emissary vein. Runs in an S-bend from the middle line to the upper orbital border in a bony vascular canal in the lower medial third of the frontal bone, usually unilateral, rarely bilateral. A vascular connection between the superior sagittal sinus and the orbital veins
6,6,6 Granular fovea (Pacchoni cavity)
6*,6* Parietal foramina permagna. Rare hereditary ossification anomalies, parasagittally in the dorsal third of the skull bones, also carrying the parietal emissary veins. This is to be distinguished from frontal bone atrophy, which is usually symmetrical but can be unilateral (trauma, lacunae, ossification)
7 Calcification in a Pacchioni cavity
8 Sulcus of the transverse sinus near the confluens sinuum. Occasionally also with calcification layering in the cerebellar tentorium
9 Calcified choroidal plexus. The result of chronic plexus neuritis, occasionally after toxoplasmosis (triad: hydrocephalus, chorioretinopathy, cerebral calcification)
10 Squamous suture. Between the frontal and temporal bones, best seen on sagittal radiograph. Can be mistaken for a fracture in sagittal radiograph. Laterally only visible in child's skull
11 Suture bones on summit of lambdoid suture
12 Mental foramen. Can be mistaken for a cyst or granuloma in the region of the deep-lying exit of the mental artery
13 Mandibular angle with projecting masseteric tuberosity

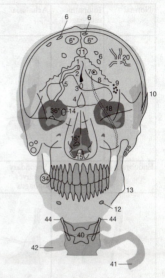

14 Calcified internal carotid artery (orthograde projection)
15 Teeth. If there is failure of synostosis with the corpus axis around the 5th year, leaving a separated tooth, the horizontal fissure must not be mistaken for a fracture.
15* Unclear apophyseal-like bony image on the tooth apex
18 Diploic occipital vein. Can be mistaken for an asymmetric fracture
20 Brechet's vein constellation, formed by diploic cranial veins
34 Retained tooth
36* Exostosis-like arch of the upper petrous bone
40 Split spinal process
41 Cervical rib
42 Great costal process
43 Laterally projecting transverse process
44,44 Calcium deposit in thyroid cartilage

(After Grashey, R. and Birkner, R. (1964))

## MEMORIX SURGERY

## Typical esophageal appearances

| Normal | Idiopathic esophageal spasm | Achalasia | Stenosis from esophagitis | Esophageal carcinoma | Carcinoma of cardia |
|---|---|---|---|---|---|
|  |  |  |  |  |  |

| Endobrachyesophagus | Secondary brachyes-ophagus | Ulcer at the epithelial transition line (frequent). Barrett's ulcer in endo-brachyesophagus (rare) |
|---|---|---|
|  |  |  |

## Abdominal survey

| Upper ileum ileus | Lower ileum ileus | Colon ileus |
|---|---|---|
|  |  |  |

Uniform fluid levels → paralytic ileus<br>Varying fluid levels → mechanical obstruction

## RADIOLOGICAL DIAGNOSIS

## Joint spaces: arthritis

### Joint spaces
**Normal width of joint space shown radiologically**
(from Thurn, P. and Bucheler, E. (1982))

| | | | |
|---|---|---|---|
| Maxillary joint | 2 mm | Sacroiliac joint | 3 mm |
| Sternoclavicular joint | 3–5 mm | Symphysis | 4–6 mm |
| Vertebral joint | 2 mm | Hip joint | 4–5 mm |
| Intervertebral disc | 5 mm | Knee joint | 3–5 mm |
| Shoulder joint | 4 mm | Ankle joint | 3–4 mm |
| Elbow joint | 4 mm | Intertarsal joint | |
| Radiocarpal joint | 2–2.5 mm | Metatarsal joint | 2–2.5 mm |
| Interphalangeal joint | 1.5–2 mm | Tarsometatarsal joint | |
| Metacarpophalangeal joint | 1.5 mm | Toe joint | 1.5 mm |

### Radiological joint spaces in children

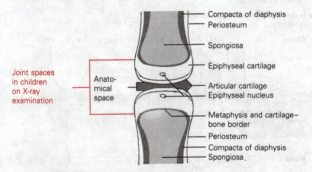

- Compacta of diaphysis
- Periosteum
- Spongiosa
- Epiphyseal cartilage
- Articular cartilage
- Epiphyseal nucleus
- Metaphysis and cartilage–bone border
- Periosteum
- Compacta of diaphysis
- Spongiosa

Joint spaces in children on X-ray examination — Anatomical space

### Radiological signs of arthritis
- Reduction in joint space, irregular incongruent joint contour
- Absorption defects, subchondral sclerosis, reactive cartilage and bone formation, production of free joint bodies
- Calcification of the joint capsule, bulging of wall

# MEMORIX SURGERY

## Normal bone development

**Normal development of important bones and epiphyses**
(From Camp, J.D. (1931))

- A     Appearance of ossification center
- U     Epiphyseal closure
- AB     Ossification apparent at birth
- Wk     Weeks
- Months     months
- Y     years
- Two-value units indicate times of ossification and epiphyseal closure (e.g. 16–25: ossification apparent at 16 years; epiphyseal closure at 25 years)

Figure for tarsal or carpal bones:
age (in years) of X-ray-visible calcification

Figure for cartilagenous union:
age (in years) at ossification

**There is considerable individual variation in every age group**

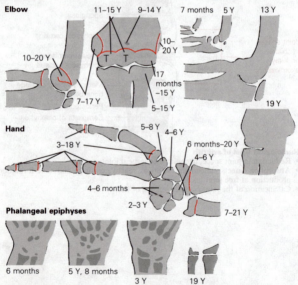

32

# RADIOLOGICAL DIAGNOSIS

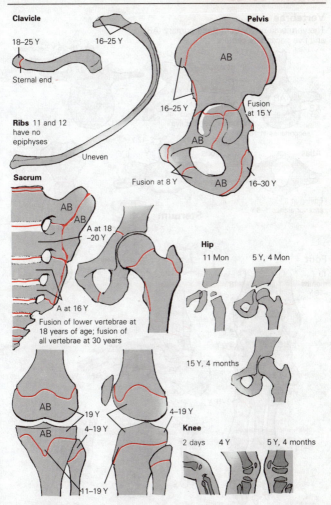

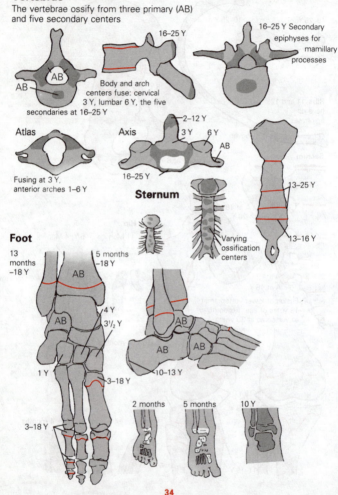

## RADIOLOGICAL DIAGNOSIS

## Bones of the wrist

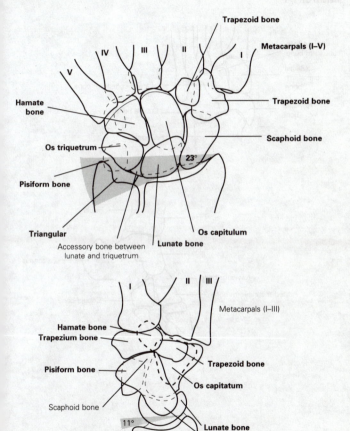

# MEMORIX SURGERY

## Bones of the foot

**Metatarsals I–V**

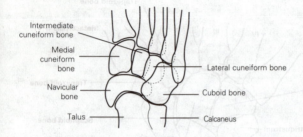

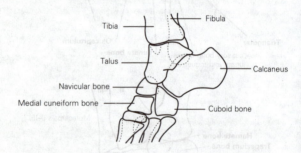

# RADIOLOGICAL DIAGNOSIS

## Preparation for specific radiological examinations

### Contrast radiography

- Thyroid radio-iodine X-ray examination: avoid giving any iodine-containing material for at least 4 weeks before the examination to avoid blocking of the iodine mechanism
- Before other contrast radiography (e.g. joints, kidney) block the thyroid with 50 droplets of perchlorate
  Leave an interval of at least 2 days between two consecutive radiocontrast examinations

### Computed tomography (CT)

- No preliminary preparation is needed for cranial CT
- Oral administration of gastrointestinal contrast material is necessary before abdominal CT
- The ileum: 1000 ml of 2% Gastrografin in solution given by mouth
- The colon: Gastrografin 2% given rectally in the CT room or orally as 1000 ml 2% Gastrografin 24 hours before the examination
- Administration of intravenous contrast material can cause nephrotoxicity
- Metallic implants (e.g. hip prostheses in pelvic CT) can cause artifacts
- NPO after midnight for all IV infusion. CT scans as the contrast material may cause vomiting

### Angiography

- The patient must be fasting for the examination, but at the same time should be well hydrated (intravenous fluid)
- Control the coagulation status and the renal function (contrast materials in dosages over 2–3 ml/kg are nephrotoxic)
- No preliminary endoscopic examination to be carried out. The giving of flatulence-producing medication beforehand may cause considerable gas artifact, as well as socially embarrassing effects

### Venography

- No special preparation required.

### Magnetic Resonance Imaging (MRI)

- No metal-containing implant
- No pacemaker present
- No aneurysm clips or metallic heart valves

## MEMORIX SURGERY

## Radiological tissue densities: Hounsfield units (HU)

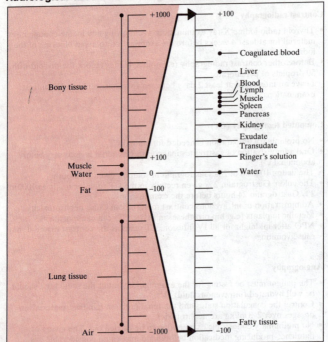

| Tissue | Value (HU) | Scatter width (HU) | Liquids | Value (HU) |
|---|---|---|---|---|
| Bones (compact) | >250 | | Blood (coagulated) | 80 ± 10 |
| Bones (spongy) | 130 ± 100 | | Blood | |
| Thyroid | 70 ± 10 | | (whole venous blood) | 55 ± 5 |
| Liver | 65 ± 5 | 45–75 | Plasma | 27 ± 2 |
| Muscle | 45 ± 5 | 35–50 | Exudate (>30 g EW/l) | >18 ± 2 |
| Spleen | 45 ± 5 | 35–55 | Transudate | |
| Lymph | 45 ± 10 | 40–60 | (<30 g EW/l) | <18 ± 2 |
| Pancreas | 40 ± 10 | 25–55 | Ringer's solution | 12 ± 2 |
| Kidney | 30 ± 10 | 20–40 | Liquor | ~10 |
| Fatty tissue | −90 ± 5 | −80−(−110) | | |

(After Wegener, O.H. (1981))

# RADIOLOGICAL DIAGNOSIS

## Magnetic Resonance Imaging

### Fundamental principles of magnetic resonance (MR)

### A spectroscopic technique in the investigation of the chemical composition of tissue

Various anatomic nuclei (e.g. hydrogen nucleus) possess a magnetic moment which, when placed in a magnetic field, aligns parallel or anti-parallel with the magnetic field lines. In clinical magnetic resonance imaging (MRI), the patient is placed in a magnetic field with field strength between 0.3 and 1.5 Tesla. The precessing hydrogen nuclei (via radiofrequency radiation stimulation and subsequent relaxation) ultimately allow the production of radiofrequency (RF) signals. The frequency of these signals is dependent upon the intensity of the magnetic field, so that (through local application of magnetic field gradients) during repeated stimulation of the nuclear signals, a good deal of local measurable information can be extracted and reconstructed for visual record via the Fourier transformation method. In the resultant acquired image, the signal intensity of the different tissues is dependent upon: (1) the two relaxation time constants ($T_1$- and $T_2$-times); (2) the repetition time (TR); (3) the echo time (TE); and (4) the stimulating angle.

Multiple techniques (pulse sequences) are used in MRI to produce optimal images. These may be divided into two main groups: (1) conventional spin–echo sequences; and (2) rapid pulse sequences (generally gradient echo sequences). Pictures of separate sections can be taken within 1 second, or of several sections in a considerably shorter period of time than with conventional techniques. In clinical application, $T_1$- or $T_2$-weighted images can be acquired using both conventional and rapid techniques. The degree of weighting of the acquired image depends upon the choice of TE/TR. In '$T_1$-weighted' images, most pathological processes (inflammation, edema, fluid) are represented by decreased signal intensity with respect to the surrounding healthy tissues. $T_2$-weighted images are more sensitive in detecting pathology; however, resolution of the images is usually reduced with respect to $T_1$-weighted images, which reveal greater anatomic detail.

## Advantages over CT

- Ability to directly acquire images in multiple planes (axial, sagittal, coronal, and oblique)
- Improved soft tissue contrast and lesion conspicuity

## Disadvantages

- Higher cost
- Longer scan time (which newer technique will shorten)

## Indications

- For the detection and characterization of suspected intracranial or intraspinal pathology (tumor or inflammatory processes, vascular malformations, cerebrovascular diseases, etc.), without artifact interference from adjacent cortical bone
- For the detection and characterization of pathology in the thorax, abdomen, and musculoskeletal system
- Concomitant injections of paramagnetic contrast material allow the determination of possible blood–brain barrier disruption and/or vascularization

## Contraindications

- The coincident presence of a cardiac pacemaker
- The presence of ferromagnetic foreign bodies, adjacent to vital structures (such as vascular aneurysm clips, metallic foreign bodies within the eye, metallic heart valves)

## Additional MR applications

- Magnetic resonance angiography (MRA) demonstrates arterial and venous structures without the use of contrast material
- Magnetic resonance spectroscopy (MRS) demonstrates metabolic changes within organs and/or pathological processes

## RADIOLOGICAL DIAGNOSIS

**MRI of the vertebral column (thoracolumbar junction)**
with sagittal stratum orientation, in $T_1$-weighted image mode, is demonstrated.

### Example

Intraspinal ependymoma (indicated by the broad arrows) before (a) and after (b) intravenous injection of paramagnetic contrast material. This causes a distinct elevation of the tumor signal. The accompanying cystic formations (angled arrow) and the spinal cord (smaller arrow) show no take-up of the contrast material.

(a)

(b)

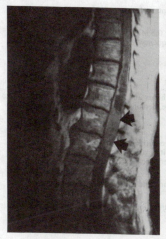
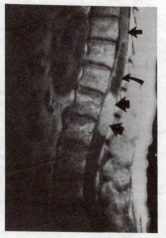

# MEMORIX SURGERY

## Fundamentals and indications

### Basic physical concepts
Ultrasound: utilizes mechanical energy in the form of sound waves
Piezoelectrical effect: conversion of mechanical to electrical energy through crystal oscillation (e.g. from quartz crystals)
Reciprocal electrical effect: conversion from electrical to mechanical energy
Acoustic impedance: material constants, defined as products of dense sound transmission velocity waves, produce different acoustic impedances, reflection, inflection, and dispersion on anatomic surface borders

### Frequencies:
Abdomen and thorax: 2.5–5 MHz; neck, joints, soft tissues, breast and vessels: 5 MHz; endosonography: 7.5 MHz

The deeper the tissue examined, the higher the MHz required
The sonic head distance also affects the frequency (e.g. the pancreas requires 3.5 MHz, the shoulder 7.5 MHz)

### Indications for emergency sonography
1. Multiple trauma
2. Cerebral trauma
3. Blunt thoracic trauma: to exclude hemothorax and hemopericardium
4. Blunt abdominal trauma: visceral damage, demonstration of blood and free fluid
5. Acute abdomen

### Endosonography
Examination of the rectal wall: maximum 6 mm thick, sound frequency 7.5 MHz; preoperative tumor staging in association with extracorporeal sonography for preoperative estimate of the surgery required (local excision, anterior resection, abdominoperineal excision) in rectal cancer.

Transrectal (endorectal) ultrasound of the prostate is useful for the evaluation of prostate cancer.

Endovaginal ultrasound may be used in conjunction with transabdominal ultrasound in evaluation of ectopic pregnancy.

## Ultrasound of internal organs

| Organ | | Pathological changes |
|---|---|---|
| Liver | Size: transverse: to 16 cm sagittal: to 15 cm, portal vein 11 mm, homologous echo, sharply delineated pointed liver lobes, intrahepatic portal vein branches, bordered, liver veins unbordered | **Circumscribed changes:**<br>– Solid: tumor, focal nodular hyperplasia (FNH), adenoma, metastases, fatty degeneration, hemangioma<br>– Liquid: dysontogenetic cysts, echinococcus, biloma, aneurysm, abscess, intra-abdominal free fluid, hematoma<br>**Diffuse changes**<br>– Hepatomegaly of various etiology, e.g. fatty infiltration, inflammations, congestive right heart failure or Budd–Chiari syndrome, portal hypertension (portal vein dilated and splenomegaly), cholestasis |
| Gallbladder | Length: 11 cm; width, 3 cm; wall, 3 mm; bile duct: ≤7mm<br>Well defined, no central echo, contracted postprandially, sometimes septated | **Central changes**<br>Stones, sludge, empyema (emphysema), hydrops<br>**Wall changes:** Polyps, tumors, inflammatory thickening<br>Other: Akinetic condition, e.g. cyst closure, positional changes before liver puncture<br>**Bile ducts:** Dilatation of the extrahepatic ducts by stones or tumor (Klatskin tumor). Similar investigation in enlargement of the head of the pancreas and in portal vein thrombosis<br>Physiological dilatation after cholecystectomy. Differential diagnosis of icterus |
| Pancreas | Size: head: 2.5–3 cm<br>Body: 1–1.5 cm, tail 2–2.5 cm<br>Pancreatic duct: 1.3 mm<br>Central structure: splenic vein in epigastric transverse view; homogeneous echogenicity | **Circumscribed changes:**<br>– Solid: head, body and caudal tumors<br>– Fluid: Dysontogenetic cysts, pseudocysts, abscesses (wall thickness of pseudocyst before cystojejunostomy: 3–4 mm)<br>**Diffuse changes:** Pancreatitis, necrosis, fat deposits, progress check<br>Other: Pancreatic duct dilatation, gall stones, checking cause of icterus contusion and rupture of pancreas by blunt abdominal trauma, accompanying reaction in the form of splenomegaly or left-sided pleural effusion |
| Spleen | Size: 4 × 7 × 11 cm<br>(thickness × width × length)<br>Convex–concave organ: homogeneous echogenicity, accessory spleen | Splenomegaly of varying etiology (diseases of the local lymph system)<br>**Circumscribed changes:**<br>– Solid: Infarct, tumors, metastases<br>– Fluid: cysts, abscesses<br>Other: rupture of spleen with free intra-abdominal fluid effusion in Morrison's pouch (subhepatic) |

| Organ | | Pathological changes |
|---|---|---|
| Kidneys | Size: 6 × 5 × 11 cm (width × thickness × length); same investigation for contralateral side calyx parenchyma relation 1:1–1.6 Well-defined pelvis | Obstruction: branching, dilated, anechoic centrally, stones above 3–4 mm visible **Circumscribed changes:** Tumors, organized hematomas, cysts, post-contusion hematoma Also: preoperative for transabdominal procedures in abdomen and pelvis (e.g. rectum) for position and check on anomalies, abscess, acute renal failure (inversion of the cortex–parenchyma proportion), transplantant retention; the ureter is normally barely visible |
| Adrenals | Length 2–7 cm, width 1.5–4 cm Not always well outlined, on the renal summit | Cysts, adenomas (if borders well-defined can be seen at below 3 cm) Metastases, e.g. from bronchial carcinoma |
| Urinary bladder | Resting content: normal <50 ml after spontaneous micturition Breadth × height × length – 0.52 Relevant for pelvic surgery | Space-occupying masses, stones in bladder, foreign bodies, papillomas, diverticulum of bladder, investigation of postoperative anuria |
| Prostate | Size: 4 × 3 × 4 cm, lies subvesically, well defined, the bladder not deformed | Tumors, adenomas, calcification, inflammations, bladder wall elevation, infiltration by rectal malignancy |
| Large abdominal vessels | Aorta: diameter 2.5 cm inferior vena cava, caliber oscillates with inspiration (↑) and expiration (↓) | Aneurysms (larger than 3 cm), calcification, retroperitoneal masses (between aorta and vertebral column – normal distance: 5 mm) Venous thickening, e.g. in lymph nodes, normally not seen Raised central venous pressure in deficient expiratory excursion |
| Thyroid | Size of a thyroid lobe: length, 4–7 cm; depth, 1–2 cm; width at isthmus, 1–3 cm Volume: 15–20 ml Homogeneous echo, well-defined outline in paratrachea | **Diffuse changes:** Diffuse struma, Hashimoto's thyroiditis, Graves' disease, Riedel's struma **Circumscribed changes** Solid: adenoma, carcinoma, hemorrhagic cyst Fluid: cyst, abscess (enclosed air) |
| Thorax | | Sonographically demonstrable pleural effusion of varying etiology over 50 ml Thoracic wall tumors, basal atelectasis |
| Breast | | Differentiation of solid and cystic processes |

## Ultrasound of joints and soft tissues

| Joint/tissue | | Pathological changes |
|---|---|---|
| Shoulder | Frequency: 5–7.5 MHz<br>sonic head position: dorsal: horizontal/vertical<br>lateral: horizontal/vertical<br>ventral: horizontal/vertical | Rupture and degeneration of the rotary cuff<br>Bankart and Hill–Sachs lesion after shoulder dislocation<br>Joint effusion<br>Bursitis<br>Arthroses<br>Instability<br>Acromioclavicular subluxation |
| Hip | Frequency: 5 MHz<br>Sonic head position: vertical, over the femoral head | Joint effusion<br>Hip-joint luxation and subluxation<br>Slipped epyphysis<br>Fluid in bursa<br>Postoperative effusion |
| Knee | Frequency: 5–7.5 MHz<br>Sonic head position: medial, lateral, dorsal<br>Vertically, over the knee joint | Joint effusion<br>Degenerative and acute meniscus injury<br>Meniscus thickening<br>Cruciate ligament injury<br>Degenerative and fresh patellar tendon lesions<br>Quadriceps tendon lesions<br>Fluid in bursa |
| Soft tissues;<br>muscles,<br>tendons | Frequency: 5–7.5 MHz<br>Sonic head position: vertical for tendons<br>transverse for muscle | Cysts<br>Solid processes<br>Tears of muscle fibers<br>Tendon rupture<br>Paratendinous thickening<br>Periosteal thickening |

# Shock

**Definition:** Peripheral circulatory failure

**Symptoms:** Tachycardia
Cold, perspiring, pale skin (extremities, periphery)
Low blood pressure, decrease in blood pressure amplitude
Dyspnea
Low urine output
Disturbances of consciousness

---

Shock Index: $\dfrac{\text{Pulse rate}}{\text{Systolic blood pressure}}$

A value >1 indicates the presence of shock
The higher the shock index, the greater the required volume replacement
Replace fluids carefully to avoid cardiogenic shock!

---

**Classification of shock**

| | | |
|---|---|---|
| **Hypovolemic** | Volume loss | Exogenous blood, plasma, fluid or electrolyte loss, endogenous extravasation |
| **Cardiogenic** | Failure of pump function | Cardiac infarct, cardiac arrhythmias, intracardiac obstruction, cardiac failure |
| **Distributive** Higher/normal resistance | Increase in venous volume content | Hypodynamic, later septic shock, autonomic block, spinal shock, overdosage of medication or drugs |
| Lowered resistance | Arteriovenous shunt | Pneumonia, peritonitis, abscess |
| **Obstructive** | Extracardiac obstruction | Obstructed vena cava, constrictive pericarditis (pericardial tamponade) |

(From Braunwald et al. (1992))

## EMERGENCIES AND ANESTHESIA

## Positioning

| Unconscious (spontaneous respiration not intubated) | Conscious |
|---|---|
| 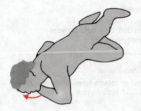<br><br>Stable lateral position | **Cerebral trauma** (Trunk raised, head in mid-position for lowering of cerebral pressure)<br>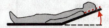<br><br>**Dyspnea** (Trunk elevated, legs resting horizontally; for cardiac failure, pulmonary edema, bronchial asthma)<br>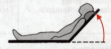<br><br>**Thoracic trauma** (Trunk elevated, lying on injured side)<br>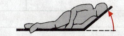<br><br>**Abdominal trauma** (Lying on back with relaxed abdominal wall, knees pulled up (knee roll) and raised head (pillow))<br>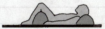<br><br>**Vertebral column trauma** (Lying flat on a vacuum mattress or flat underlay. Transport under traction with steady body position)<br>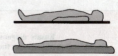 |

# MEMORIX SURGERY

## Resuscitation

**EMERGENCY CALL:** Where?
What?
How many casualties?

| Diagnosis | Immediate life-saving measures |
|---|---|
| **Unconsciousness**<br>Patient does not respond to calling and is insensitive to pain | **A: Clear airways**<br>1. Esmarch's maneuver<br>   head extended, chin held forward<br>2. Foreign-body removal |
| **No respiration**<br>No respiratory effort<br>No respiratory movements<br>Cyanosis | **B: Artificial respiration**<br>Mouth-to-nose or mouth-to-mouth respiration<br>Frequency: 12–15 breaths/min |
| **Circulatory arrest**<br>Pulse not palpable<br>(try carotid or femoral pulse) | **C: Cardiopulmonary resuscitation (CPR)**<br>External chest compression<br>Frequency: 80–100/min combined with artificial respiration |

| | **Chest compression** |
|---|---|
| Pressure point: | Area between middle and lower third of the sternum |
| Technique: | Arms extended: shoulders of helper vertically over patient |
| Goal: | To approximate the sternum 4 cm to the vertebral column in the adult patient |

| | **Cardiopulmonary resuscitation** |
|---|---|
| **One helper:** | 2 initial breaths; thorax compression/respiration = 15:2 |
| **Two helpers:** | 2 initial breaths; thorax compression/respiration = 5:1 |

**Note**
**Ensure diagnosis – treat immediately**
**Rapid treatment increases the chances for successful resuscitation**

## EMERGENCIES AND ANESTHESIA

Extended immediate life-saving measures on arrival of resuscitation team

**Oxygen**  **Intubation**
**ECG**  **Defibrillation**
**Insert intravenous line**  **Medication**

**Circulatory failure**
↓
Stimulation (see Resuscitation I)
↓
**ECG findings**

| Asystole | Ventricular fibrillation | Electromechanical dissociation |
|---|---|---|
| • | Defibrillation with increasing energy | |
| • | CPR, if no pulse | |
| • | Intravenous therapy | |
| • | Adrenaline 1 : 10 000<br>5–10 ml = 0.5–1 mg | Adrenaline 1 : 10 000<br>or endotracheal 1–2 mg |
| • | Intubation ($F_{IO_2} = 1.0$) | • |
| • | Defibrillation to 360 Joule | • |
| • | Lidocaine 50–100 mg | • |
| • | $NaHCO_3$ after<br>return of heart beat | • |
| Pacemaker<br>indication check | | Pacemaker<br>indication check |

**Note**
After each procedure, check pulse rate and rhythm, repeat cardiopulmonary resuscitation if necessary

## MEMORIX SURGERY

## Trauma: assessment and management

**First overview**

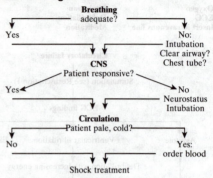

**Shock treatment**

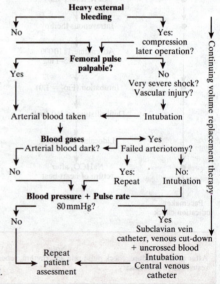

(Modified from Tscherne, H. et al. (1988))

## EMERGENCIES AND ANESTHESIA

**Check-up**

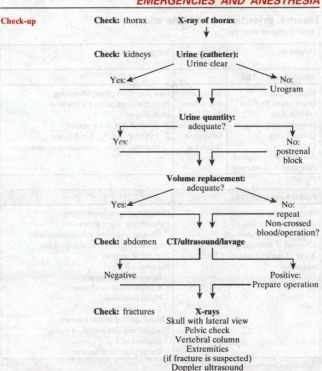

(From Tscherne, H. *et al.* (1988))

## MEMORIX SURGERY

## Trauma: priorities in multiple injury
(After Tscherne et al. 1987)

| Diagnosis | Acute measures | Surgical measures |
|---|---|---|
| **Acute phase (1–3 h)** | | |
| Vital functions<br>Orientation, physical examination<br>Neurostatus (Glasgow-Coma Scale)<br>Chest X-ray<br>Abdominal ultrasound<br>Assessment of severity<br>CT | Secure IV access lines, fluid replacement<br>Intubation<br>Breathing | First operative-phase life-saving immediate operation for massive hemorrhage<br>1. Internal (e.g. liver, spleen)<br>2. External (e.g. open pelvic and shoulder injury, penetrating wounds) |
| **Primary phase (3–72 h)** | | |
| More specific laboratory and circulatory diagnosis<br>Exclude vascular damage<br>Urogram if hematuria is present<br>X-ray of skeletal system if fracture is suspected | | Closed and open brain injury<br>Parenchyma organ injury (thorax, abdomen, retroperitoneum)<br>Progress of spinal cord compression<br>Eye, facial injuries<br>Peripheral injuries:<br>  Injury of large vessels<br>  Compartment syndrome<br>  Open fractures<br>  Open joint injuries<br>Closed shaft of femur fracture<br>Fracture and dislocation of pelvis<br>  Fracture of leg<br>  Other peripheral injuries |
| **Secondary/regeneration phase (3–10 days)** | | |
| Monitoring of stable cardiopulmonary function<br>Early recognition of septic complications | | Definitive fracture treatment (mid-face, frontobasal, mandible, upper extremities, joint reconstruction)<br>Eradication of septic foci<br>Reconstruction of large soft tissue defects<br>Evacuation of hematomas |
| **Tertiary phase (after day 8)** | | |
| Early recognition of septic complications and organ failure | | Meticulous soft tissue reconstruction<br>Plastic repair of amputation stump<br>All postponed secondary operations |

# EMERGENCIES AND ANESTHESIA

## Tracheostomy

Skin incision

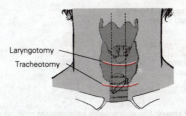

Midline incision between vertical veins and strap muscles (sternohyoid and sternothyroid)

Displacing the thyroid gland
Transecting the isthmus

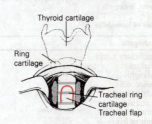

Tracheostomy

Forming a caudally based tracheal flap by an arched incision through the 2 and 3 tracheal cartilage rings
Fixation by suture of the tracheal flap to the caudal skin margin

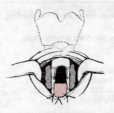

Insertion and fixation of the tracheostomy tube with obturator

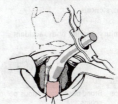

# Gastrointestinal (GI) bleeding

## Causes of upper GI bleeding
(Morgan and Clamp)

| | |
|---|---|
| Ulcer | 36.0% |
| Hemorrhagic gastritis | 22.1% |
| Esophageal varices | 13.4% |
| Gastric erosions | 6.9% |
| Esophagitis | 4.1% |
| Carcinoma | 2.6% |
| Mallory–Weiss syndrome | 2.4% |
| No diagnosis | 6.5% |

**Systematic causes:** Blood dyscrasias, anticoagulant medication, uremia, autoimmune diseases, leukemia

## Causes of hemobilia

| Intrahepatic | Extrahepatic |
|---|---|
| Angiobiliary fistula | Aneurysm (hepatic, splenic arteries) |
| Ascarides | Cholangitis |
| Cholangitis | Cholelithiasis |
| Echinococcus | Bile duct tumor |
| Cholelithiasis | Tumor of pancreas |
| Hepatic abscess | Pancreatitis |
| Rupture of liver | |
| Tumor of liver | |

## Differential diagnosis of lower GI bleeding

**Anomalies**
Endometriosis, Meckel's diverticulum
Angiodysplasia

**Inflammatory**
Crohn's disease, colitis (ulcerative, radiation, bacterial, toxic, tuberculous colitis), diverticulitis, proctitis, ulcer, enteritis, fistula, fissure

**Mechanical**
Invagination, stenosis

**Trauma**
Iatrogenic injury, foreign body, accident

**Tumor**
Carcinoma, polyp, polyposis, adenomatosis, fibroma, lipoma, neuroma, sarcoma, metastasis

**Vascular**
Hemangioma, angioenteral fistula, mesenteric infarct, hemorrhoids, telangiectases, varicosities

**Systemic**
Blood dyscrasias, autoimmune disease, uremia, anticoagulant medication, leukemia

**Diagnosis**
Rectal examination
Proctoscopy
Coloscopy
Angiography
Basic diagnosis of bleeding disorders (see p. 19)

Stalked polyps    Broad-based polyps    Villous polyps

Types of intestinal polyp

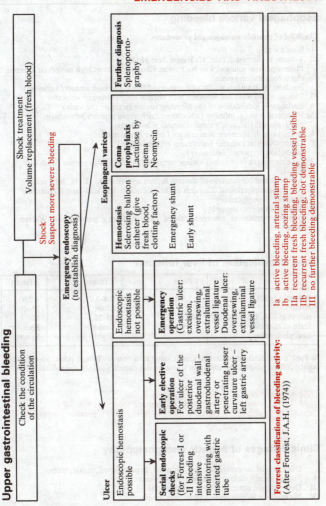

## Esophageal varices bleeding

#### Checklist of possible management procedures

1. Start i.v. drip
2. Volume replacement (aim CVP over 5 cm $H_2O$)
   Plasma-protein solution, low Na human albumin; caution: high molecular Dextran alerts coagulation system
   Fresh blood transfusions (stored preserved blood has high ammonia content)
3. Evacuate and wash out stomach with normal temperature or ice water
4. Endoscopic localization of the bleeding source (sclerose the varix)
5. Vasopressin as i.v. infusion (advantage: fairly rapid primary hemostasis; disadvantage: frequently cardiovascular side effects)
6. Sengstaken–Blakemore, if necessary (under X-ray control)
   Linton–Nachlas catheter (maximum retention 12 h)
   Intubation (expertise necessary)
7. Give neomycin (4–6 g/day) and/or lactulose 100 g/day, high enema (wash out blood)
8. Any required substitution of clotting factors and vitamins (K, $B_1$, folic acid)
9. Adequate correction of disorders in the electrolyte and acid–base equilibrium (caution: hypoglycemia)
10. Angiography (portography)
11. Definitive treatment [emergency shunt, early shunt (e.g. portocaval or Warren shunt)]


## Child classification of liver function

|  | 1 Point | 2 Points | 3 Points |
|---|---|---|---|
| Albumin (g/dl) | >3.5 | 3.4–3.0 | <3.0 |
| Ascites | – | Little | Much |
| Bilirubin (µmol/l) | 34 | 35–51 | 51 |
| State of nutrition | Very good | Good | Poor |
| Encephalopathy | – | Slight | Severe |

In Pugh's classification the actual Quick value is increased (70%, 1 point; 50–60%, 2 points; 50%, 3 points): the nutrition status on the contrary falls in the valuation


Child A (5–8 points)     Patient requires operation
Child B (7–11 points)     Patient can be operated (operative risk: 10%)
Child C (10–12 points)    Patient should not be operated (operative risk: high)


## Clinical stages of hepatic encephalopathy

I     Disorders of concentration and attention, hyperreflexed, ataxia, tremor
II    Fading speech, delayed reaction to questions
III   Delayed pain reaction, clonic contractions
IV   No reaction to questioning or to pain, coma

# EMERGENCIES AND ANESTHESIA

## Thermal and chemical burns

**Criteria for transfer to a burn center** (American Burn Association)

- 20% TBSA 2nd or 3rd degree burns
- 10% TBSA 2nd or 3rd degree burns in patients <10 or >50 years old
- 5% TBSA 3rd degree burn
- 2nd or 3rd degree burns to face, hands, feet, major joints, perineum, genitalia
- Chemical burn
- Inhalation injury
- Electrical injury, lightning
- Burns associated with major trauma
- Burns associated with co-morbid factors (age, chronic alcoholism, drug abuse, heart disease, compromised immune system, etc.)

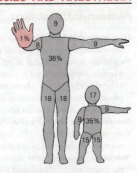

### Burn size (% total body surface area – TBSA)

- Rough estimate by rule of 9's
- Palmar surface roughly represents 1% TBSA
- Major adjustments are necessary for different age groups (adult–child)

### Burn wound depth

- amount of tissue destruction depends on temperature (>40°C) and exposure time
- often deeper in children and older persons

| Degree | Involvement | Symptoms | Treatment | Prognosis |
|---|---|---|---|---|
| 1st | Epidermis | Redness, pain, swelling | External cooling, anti-inflammatory drugs | Complete restitution of skin |
| Superficial 2nd | Superficial dermis | Blister formation, blanching of skin | Local wound care | Complete restitution of skin |
| Deep 2nd | Deep dermis | Blister formation, reduced pain, hair follicles intact | Local wound care, surgical débridement and grafting probably necessary | Incomplete restitution, hypertrophic scarring possible |
| 3rd | All layers of skin | No pain, no blanching, hair can be pulled out easily | Surgical débridement and grafting | Incomplete restitution, hypertrophic scarring possible |

## Assessment/treatment

**History, physical** (immunization including tetanus, risk factors like pre-existing immunodeficiency, GI ulcers, alcohol or drug abuse, others)

**Respiratory status** (suspicion of inhalation injury when injury occurred in closed quarters, especially in the presence of vinyl, burned nasal hair, carbon particles in pharynx, or hoarseness – **bronchoscopy is diagnostic gold standard**, humidified oxygen by facemask, intubation, escharotomy)

**Associated conditions** (i.e. fractures, pregnancy, others)

**Nasogastric tube** (intermittent low suction) for burns >20% TBSA

**Foley catheter** for burns >15% or for exact recording of intake and output (I&O), permanent monitoring of urinary output

**Nutritional support** (as early as possible, oral feeding, nasoenteric tube feeding, total parenteral nutrition associated with 10–20% increased rate of sepsis)

**Circumferential** burn (watch for early signs of compartment syndrome, Doppler and/or laser–Doppler exam, determine direct compartment pressures, **good capillary refill is not reliable!**, maintain affected extremities elevated, enzymatic or surgical escharotomy or fasciotomy may be indicated)

Baseline laboratory studies (hematocrit, BUN, electrolytes, CO, arterial blood gases, urine and sputum specimens for analysis, culture and sensitivity, and others, chest X-ray, ECG)

Prognosis is determined by burn size, age, and presence of inhalation injury and major risk factors

## Fluid management

Decision about formal fluid resuscitation versus administration of maintenance fluids

Baxter or Parkland formula: 4 ml Ringer's lactate × body weight (kg) × % TBSA burn for the first 24 hours starting at the time of injury; half of the calculated fluid over the first 8 hours following the burn, half of the calculated fluid over the next 16-hour period

I.v. fluids to maintain urine output >0.5 ml (adults) – 1 ml (children) /kg body weight

Pulse <120/min (adults) – 140/min (children)

In large burns and/or patients with risk factors (i.e. heart disease) monitoring of fluid management by pulmonary wedge pressures (Swan–Ganz catheter)

Starting at 18–24 hours after the injury 0.5 ml plasma (colloid, fresh frozen plasma) × % TBSA burn × kg body weight over period of 4–8 hours, may be supplemented by free water plus electrolytes as needed to maintain urine output and normal sodium

## EMERGENCIES AND ANESTHESIA

## Wound management

Photo documentation
Cleanse, débride, and cover burn wound (protection against desiccation and contamination, if indicated – antimicrobials like sulfadiazine or mafenide acetate)
Maintain elevation of burned extremities and burned face
Wound closure by split thickness skin autograft, cultured epidermis and/or dermis, allograft (i.e. cadaver skin), xenograft (i.e. pigskin), artificial skin. The greater the dermal remnant of the débrided wound, and the greater the dermal content of the autograft, the better the functional result of the burn wound
Functionally (hands, fingers, important joints) or cosmetic (face) important areas should be grafted first
Intensive physical and occupational therapy, splinting if necessary (elbow extension, resting hand, 'pancake') for early restoration of normal function

## Inhalation injury

Causes chemical injury to alveolar basement membrane and pulmonary edema
May present in three stages: acute pulmonary distress, pulmonary edema, bronchopneumonia
Bronchoscopy for initial diagnosis and treatment (removal of carbonaceous and mucous materials)
Many require serial therapeutic bronchoscopies

## Complications

|  | Cause | Prophylaxis | Treatment |
|---|---|---|---|
| Infection | Burn wound sepsis<br>Pneumonia<br>Urinary tract infection<br>Abdominal process<br>Any catheter | Early enteral feeding<br>Frequent changes of i.v. sites | Specific antibacterials |
| GI bleeding | Stress | $H_2$ blocker, antacids<br>Monitor gastric pH | Conservative if feasible (see p. 54) |
| Lack of graft take | Insufficient débridement<br>Infection of wound bed | Avoid causes<br>Delay autografting, if in doubt regarding proper wound bed | Treat wound infection<br>Quantitative biopsies<br>Bacterial counts $<10^5$<br>Débride all necrotic tissue |
| Hypertrophic scarring | Lack of intact dermis | Prompt and complete wound closure | Symptomatic:<br>Pressure garment<br>Local silicone sheet applications<br>Excision |
| Functional deficit | Late wound closure<br>Hypertrophic scarring | Physical/occupational therapy<br>Splinting | Surgical release, i.e. full-thickness graft or z-plasty |

## Electrical injury

High risk for initial ventricular fibrillation and delayed rhythm abnormalities
High risk for renal failure due to increased **myoglobin**, potassium, protein, toxic waste products, and others
Dependent on amperage, voltage, resistance, duration of contact, pathway through the body, type of injury (arc, direct contact)
Low voltage (<1000 volts), high voltage (>1000 volts)
Fluid requirement may be considerably higher than for thermal injuries, i.e. 9 ml/kg weight × % TBSA burn, adequate fluids are the key to avoid renal complications
Urine outputs should exceed 75–100 ml/hour, may add mannitol 12.5 g, and bicarbonate to i.v. to alkalinize urine
Monitor urine output for myoglobin until completely absent

## Chemical injury

– agent
– concentration

| Agent | Treatment |
|---|---|
| Gasoline | Burn wound care, water dilution<br>**Caution**: pulmonary complications, hepatic and renal complications |
| Hydrofluoric acid | Irrigate copiously with water, subcutaneous injection of 10% calcium gluconate<br>**Caution**: hypocalcemia, pulmonary edema, analgesics |
| Phenol | Spray water on burned areas, wipe with polyethylene glycol<br>**Caution**: renal toxicity |
| White phosphorus | Mechanical removal of all particles<br>**Caution**: ECG changes, hemoglobinemia, renal failure, avoid exposure to air, keep wound moist |
| Tar | Removal with petroleum solvents |

## Cold injury (hypothermia/frostbite)

– local (frostbite, chilblains, immersion foot, arctic willy, etc.)
  rapid rewarming, 40 °C (104 °F) water bath, wound care, infection control, bone scan to add in distinguishing of viable versus necrotic tissues, amputation, soft tissue coverage, reconstruction
– systemic (hypothermia – core temperature <34 °C)
  rapid rewarming, correction of acidosis
– severity of frostbite

| Degree | Symptoms | Treatment |
|---|---|---|
| 1st | Skin white | External rewarming, monitoring of circulation, analgesics |
| 2nd | Blisters, clear fluid | Wound care, débridement of blisters, topical antimicrobials, analgesics |
| 3rd | Blisters, dark fluid | Wound care, débridement of blisters, amputation, soft tissue coverage, reconstruction |

## EMERGENCIES AND ANESTHESIA

# Emergency pediatric surgery

### Vomiting

- Alkaline (esophagus)
- Colorless (stomach)
- Greenish (duodenum)
- Brownish (small intestine)
- Explosive (hypertrophic pyloric stenosis, upper jejunal obstruction)
- Effortless (chalasia)

### Vomiting without ileus (Potential incomplete ileus)

#### Chalasia/hiatal hernia

Symptoms: pale vomiting without effort, often of undigested food, failure to thrive, subsequent dysphagia

Diagnosis: X-rays demonstrate reflux, endoscopy, sonography, pH probe

Treatment: thicken feedings, frequent small meals, upright positioning, operation if necessary around 6–8 months of age

#### Hypertrophic pyloric stenosis

Symptoms: projectile vomiting, acid, visible gastric peristalsis, dehydration, alkalosis and electrolyte shift

Diagnosis: sonography and/or gastrointestinal intubation, barium swallow

Treatment: nasogastric tube, nil-by-mouth, and early transfer for pyloromyotomy

#### Intussusception

Symptoms: sudden cramp-like pains, with pain-free intervals of 30 minutes. Typically around age 2, vomiting and ileus visually present, bloody stool with mucus

Diagnosis: palpable cylindrical swelling in right mid-abdomen, rectal examination shows first mucus, later blood content, sonography, colon contrast enema

Treatment: attempt hydrostatic reduction by barium enema up to 48 hours if no signs of strangulated bowel or perforation

# MEMORIX SURGERY

**Vomiting with ileus**

**Duodenal atresia, annular pancreas**

Symptoms: flat abdomen, early bilious vomiting, enlarged stomach
Diagnosis: X-rays: 'double bubble' phenomenon
Treatment: nasogastric tube, nil-by-mouth, surgical correction, explore GI tract for other anomalies

**Malrotation**

Symptoms: recurrent vomiting, light green to green, often without complete bowel obstruction
Diagnosis: X-rays: little or no gas presence in the whole small intestine, barium studies helpful
Treatment: nasogastric tube, nil-by-mouth, surgical intervention

**Volvulus**

Torsion and closure of the bowel on the mesenteric root by failure of mesofixation
Symptoms: symptoms of ileus, distended abdomen, rapid deterioration
Treatment: nasogastric tube, nil-by-mouth, emergency transfer for surgery

**Jejunal atresia**

Symptoms: green and brown emesis, palpable dilated tender loops, abdomen distended above the level of the atresia
Diagnosis: tinkling or absent peristalsis, X-ray: several very distended bowel loops
Treatment: nasogastric tube with continuous suction, danger of perforation, emergency transfer for surgery

**Meconium ileus**

Viscous and thickened meconium occupies the distal ileum, often the first sign of cystic fibrosis
Symptoms: distended abdomen, green emesis, no meconium passed
Diagnosis: X-ray: air distention, fluid levels, barium enema useful
Treatment: nasogastric tube, nil-by-mouth, transfer for double ileostomy and contrast washout, emergency transfer for surgery

**Incarcerated inguinal hernia**

Symptoms: palpable firm, tender swelling in the inguinal region, persistent pain, vomiting is a late sign
Diagnosis: palpation
Treatment: elevation of buttocks, attempt manipulative reduction under sedation, if irreducible correct surgically

# EMERGENCIES AND ANESTHESIA

**Ileus**

**Duplication**

Localized to mesenteric side of any segment of bowel

Symptoms: obstruction by compressing adjoining intestine, bleeding from ulceration, pain, moveable mass

Diagnosis: sonography, X-rays of limited value, diagnosis often made intraoperatively

Treatment: nasogastric tube, close inpatient monitoring, transfuse if hemodynamic compromise

**Necrosing enterocolitis**

Symptoms: abdominal distention, visible bowel loops, skin discoloration, blood in stool, other evidence of 'sepsis'

Diagnosis: decreased peristalsis, fixed loop of bowel, intraluminal air, intrahepatic air

Treatment: nasogastric tube, nil-by-mouth, i.v. antibiotics, X-rays every 6 hours, surgery in severe cases

**Hirschsprung's disease**

Symptoms: distended abdomen with green emesis, defecation problems, alternating constipation and diarrhea

Diagnosis: mass palpable, extremely tight sphincter muscle on rectal examination, X-ray shows ileus, fail to evacuate barium after enema, rectal biopsy with absent ganglion cells is diagnostic

Treatment: nasogastric tube, nil-by-mouth, surgical intervention

**Toxic megacolon/enterocolitis**

Symptoms: bloated abdomen with extreme distention of the small or large intestine, often 'septic' appearance

Diagnosis: X-ray examination shows extreme intestinal dilatation, diagnostic emptying by rectal tube of toxic bowel contents

Treatment: gastric emptying, infusion, intestinal washouts, immediate transfer for double colostomy as emergency operation

## MEMORIX SURGERY

**Breathing disorders**
Tachypnea (normal: newborn 35–40/min, 2 years 20–25/min)
Respiratory distress (retractions, abdominal breathing, nasal flaring, grunting)
Cyanosis (blue lips, nail beds)
Tachycardia (normal: newborn 140/min, child 100/min)

**Pediatric causes of respiratory distress**

Asphyxia, aspiration, hyaline membrane disease, airway obstruction, pneumonia

**Diaphragmatic hernia**

Symptoms: dyspnea soon after birth, worsened by hand bagging (forces air into stomach/intestine)
Diagnosis: peristalsis in the chest, heart and mediastinum displaced
X-rays: intestine in thorax, visible on left side
Treatment: intubation, nasogastric tube with continuous suction
Comment: Often spontaneous pneumothorax causes sudden worsening condition with mortality 50%

**Esophageal atresia**

Symptoms: saliva accumulation in mouth, aspiration pneumonia, immediate emesis of feeding
Diagnosis: nasogastric tube passage obstructed, barium swallow X-rays diagnostic
Treatment: frequent suctioning, place patient on right side, elevate upper body to minimize risk of aspiration, surgical correction
Comment: around 25% have congenital heart defect, otherwise prognosis good

**Congenital lobar emphysema**

Symptoms: severe respiratory distress in early infancy, over-inflation of various lobes
Diagnosis: examination unreliable
X-rays: hyperinflated radiolucent lobe, mediastinal shift
Treatment: intubation, surgical intervention

**Foreign-body aspiration**

Symptoms: sudden dyspnea without inflammatory signs
Diagnosis: respiratory distress with stridor, X-ray can show hyperinflation, atelectasis, or pneumonia
Treatment: intubation, bronchoscopy

**Stress pneumothorax**

Symptoms: sudden respiratory distress, begins with piercing pain
Diagnosis: absent breath sounds, X-rays show cardiac displacement
Treatment: thoracic aspiration or drainage

**Tracheal stenosis**

Symptoms: inspiratory stridor caused by tracheal compression (lymph nodes, vascular rings, tumors), or intratracheal pathology (inflammation, infection, scarring, tracheal collapse, inspirational stridor)
Diagnosis: X-rays or bronchoscopy
Treatment: intubation, tracheostomy, bronchoscopy

## EMERGENCIES AND ANESTHESIA

**Acute scrotum**

Courses of painful scrotal mass: torsion of spermatic cord, torsion of testicular appendix, trauma, epididymitis, orchitis.

| | Length of history | Redness Swelling | Thickened cord | Tenderness | Doppler sonography | Radionuclide scan | Treatment |
|---|---|---|---|---|---|---|---|
| Torsion of spermatic cord | Hours | ++ | + | Whole testis | No flow | Increased uptake | Emergency surgery |
| Torsion of appendix | Hours | + | − | Unipolar | Normal to increased flow | Normal uptake | Analgesia, anti-inflammatory agents |
| Epididymitis | Days | ++ | + | Adjacent | Increased flow | Increased uptake | Analgesia; antibiotics |

# Anesthesia: preparation

### 1. Examination

### 2. Grading the anesthetic risk

| 0 | 1 | 2 | 4 | 8 | 16 |
|---|---|---|---|---|---|
| Status | Ambulant | Emergency | | | |
| Planned operation | Urgent operation | Immediate | | | |
| Age 1–39 y | 0–1<br>Age 40–69 y | Age 70–79 y | age >80 y | | |
| Normal weight 10% | 10–30% over<br>10–15% under | 30–50% over<br>15–25% under | >50% over<br>>25% under | | |
| >6 h fasting | <6 h fasting | <1 h | | | |
| Conscious | Drowsy | Comatose | | | |
| BP stable | Hypotension | Laboratory hypertension | Fixed hypertension | Compensated shock | Decompensated shock |
| Heart healthy | Cardiac insufficiency compensated | Decreased cardiac function | Myocardial infarction <2 months | Compression failure | Decompression failure |
| Pulse rate normal | Irregular rhythm | Tachycardia; arrhythmia | VPCs | | Complete A-V block |
| Respiration normal | Dyspnea | Bronchitis | Pneumonia | Respiratory failure | |
| Renal function normal | Renal failure | Anuria; uremia | | | |
| Liver function normal | Liver failure | Hepatic coma | | | |
| Blood sugar normal | Controlled diabetes | Uncontrolled diabetes | | | |
| Electrolytes normal | Hyperkalemia >5 mmol | Hyperkalemia <3 mmol | Hyperkalemia <2.5 mmol | | |
| Hydration normal | | | Dehydration | | |
| Hb >12.5 g/dl | Hb 12.5–7.5 g/dl | Hb <7.5 g/dl | | | |
| No allergies | Allergic | | | | |
| No other disease | | Other severe disease | | | |
| Anticipated operation time <120 min | Anticipated operation time 121–180 min | Anticipated operation time >180 min | | | |
| Burns | <15%; no pulmonary | | 15–50%; burn no pulmonary | >50%; burn and/or pulmonary | >50% burn and pulmonary |
| **Risk group** | **I (0–1)** | **II (2–3)** | **III (4–7)** | **IV (8–15)** | **V (over 15)** |

The anesthetic risk is proportional to the group (I–V) and the number (0–15)

### 3. Choice of anesthetic procedure depending on the urgency and type of operation

| General anesthesia | Regional anesthesia | |
|---|---|---|
| Inhalation<br>Intubation anesthesia<br>Total intravenous anesthesia<br>Neuroleptic anesthesia | Spinal cord procedures<br>• Spinal anesthesia<br>• Epidural anesthesia<br><br>I.v. regional<br>(Bier block) | Peripheral block<br>• Infiltration anesthesia – field block<br>• Conduction anesthesia – peripheral nerve block<br>• Brachial plexus<br>• Hand block<br>• Knee block<br>• Foot block |

> **Note: peripheral block involves the least risk**
> **It is preferable to general anesthesia and spinal block**

## EMERGENCIES AND ANESTHESIA

4. **Explanation**/agreement with the patient (personal explanatory talk, written documentation)

5. **Premedication**
   Aim: relief of anxiety
   e.g. 0.3 mg/kg body weight nordazepam by mouth, at least 1 h preoperatively

6. **Further preparation**
   - Optimize the cardiopulmonary situation by elective intervention
   - Aspiration prophylaxis

   Danger: aspiration of acid gastric juice
   Recognition of dangers: ileus, ulcer, prengancy, <6 h or >12 h fasting, preoperative trauma or stress situation nicotine addict
   Management: Empty stomach, alkalize gastric juice, prevent regurgitation

### Management
(range according to the remaining time before operation)

**Emergency procedures Ileus Patient with full stomach**

Incipient ileus (Sellick's maneuver)
Aspirate gastric fluids
20 ml 0.3 M Na citrate by mouth
Metoclopromide (not with ileus)
$H_2$-antagonists

Anxiolytics
Fasting period
'Caution': nicotine

**Prophylaxis**

## Intraoperative monitoring

| Patient monitoring | Safety monitoring |
|---|---|
| ECG | Inspired oxygen concentration |
| Blood pressure | Disconnections and leakages |
| Check secretions | Respiratory pressure, blockage alarm |
| Check pulse oximeter | Pulse oximeter and end-tidal $CO_2$ |
| Pulmonary artery catheter | Nerve stimulator |
| EEG | Measure anesthetic gas concentration |

**Note:**
The **higher** the risk, the more **invasive** the monitoring
**No** monitor can replace an experienced **anesthetist**

# MEMORIX SURGERY

## Volume replacement

> Initial fluid deficit
> + maintenance needed
> + loss
> _____
> = intraoperative fluid requirement

**Basic fluid maintenance**

Adults: 2 ml/kg/h

Children: water and electrolyte requirements depend on age and stage of development:

 0–10 kg   6 ml/kg/h
 11–20 kg  4 ml/kg/h
 20 kg     2 ml/kg/h

## Intraoperative blood loss

*Danger:* Hypovolemic shock

*Treatment:* Volume replacement    Electrolyte solution
                                      Plasma expander
                                      Erythrocyte concentrate
            in consumption coagulopathy   Thrombocyte concentrate
                                      Clotting-active fresh plasma

> **Danger of infection from donated blood**

## Important: measures to avoid donor blood transfusion

**Preoperative autologous blood donation**
**Plasmaphoresis**
**Isovolemic hemodilution**
**Autologous re-transfusion**
**Intraoperative reclaimed blood transfusion**

> **Note:**
> The patient should be informed about the risks of donor blood transfusion when elective surgery is planned.
> The possibility of autotransfusion should be utilized preoperatively.

# MINIMALLY INVASIVE SURGERY

## Endoscopic surgery: fundamentals

### Advantages

Less surgical trauma
- less pain
- smaller incisions
- short postoperative gastrointestinal ileus

Low rate of wound infection (the small trochar sites reduce contamination of the abdominal wall)

Rapid mobilization and convalescence

Short hospital stay

Short period off work

Good cosmetic result

### Indications

Appendectomy
Cholecystectomy
Removal of adhesions
Explorative laparoscopy
Hernia operation
Wedge excision from liver
Second-look operation
Vagotomy

### Contraindications

- Cardiopulmonary insufficiency (raised intrathoracic pressure with established pneumoperitoneum)
- Ileus with major intestinal distention
- Perforation with peritonitis
- Malignancy of the organ treated
- Large tumors

### Assumptions

- Perfect command of conventional operative technique
- Adequate laparoscopic instruction and experience of the operator and his operative team

### Informed consent

- New surgical technique
- Requires procedural changes from conventional surgery
- Possibility of complications in laparoscopy and conventional operation
- Specific laparoscopic complications (subcutaneous emphysema, gas embolism, iatrogenic injury (vessels, hollow organs, parenchyma), coagulation injury to adjacent structures, retained foreign body (e.g. swab) in the peritoneal cavity)

## MEMORIX SURGERY

### Endoscopic surgery: techniques

**Endoscopic appendectomy**
Access sites for optical trocar (OT) and operation trochar (AT)

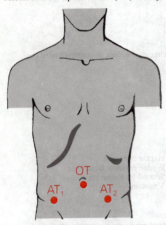

AT$_1$ Appendix extractor

AT$_2$ Manipulator, coagulation forceps, scissors, etc.

**Endoscopic cholecystectomy**
Possible access sites for optical trochar (OT) and operation trochar (AT)

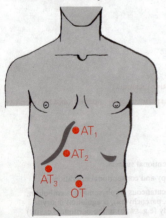

AT$_1$ (right paramedian) Holding forceps, coagulation forceps, sucker, scissors

AT$_2$ (right medioclavicular line) Holding forceps, punction cannula

AT$_3$ (right axillary line) Gallbladder extractor

# SKIN AND SOFT TISSUE SURGERY

## Langer's skin lines

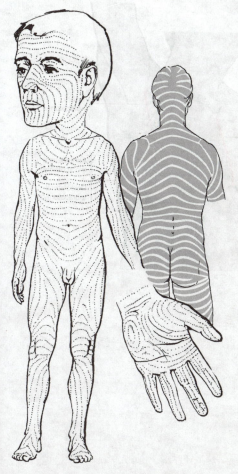

# MEMORIX SURGERY

## Common incisions

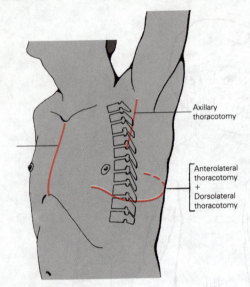

Median sternotomy

Axillary thoracotomy

Anterolateral thoracotomy
+
Dorsolateral thoracotomy

## SKIN AND SOFT TISSUE SURGERY

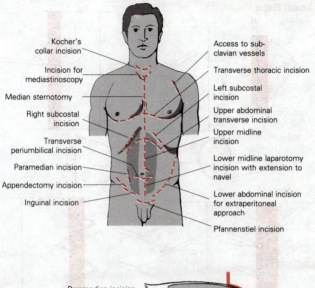

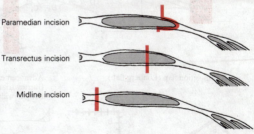

# MEMORIX SURGERY

## Local flaps

Z-plasty

V–Y-flap

Y–V-plasty

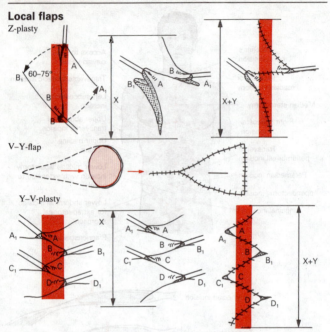

Transposition flap (Limberg flap)

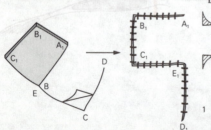

Advancement flap (×2) with four Burraw triangles
Length–width-relation of flap: <2:1!

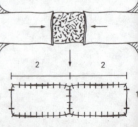

## SKIN AND SOFT TISSUE SURGERY

**Skin/flap anatomy**

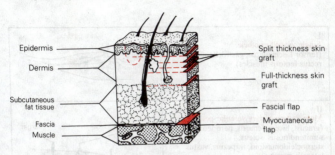

**Local and distant flaps**

|  | I Intact pedicle | II Free flap |
|---|---|---|
| (A) Random subdermal plexus blood supply | Transposition flap (Limberg)<br>Advancement flap<br>Z-plasty<br>V–Y-plasty<br>V–Y flap |  |
| (B) Fascial vascular plexus | Abdominal wall flap<br>Cross-leg flap |  |
| (C) Axial fascial blood supply | Temporal fascial<br>Dorsalis pedis<br>Groin flap<br>Tensor fascia lata flap<br>Deltoid scapular |  |
| (D) Myocutaneous or muscle alone | Latissimus dorsi flap<br>Transverse rectus muscle flap | Free latissimus dorsi |

## Mathes–Nahai classification

| | |
|---|---|
| **I**<br>Single vascular pedicle<br>(tensor fasciae latae, gastrocnemius, rectus femoris muscles) | |
| **II**<br>Main and secondary vascular pedicles<br>(gracilis, biceps femoris, peroneus, semitendinosus, soleus, sternocleidomastoid, trapezius, vastus lateralis muscles) | smaller / larger |
| **III**<br>Two main vascular pedicles<br>(gluteus maximus, rectus abdominis, serratus anterior, semimembranosus, temporalis muscles) | |
| **IV**<br>Segmental vascular pedicles<br>(sartorius, extensor digitorum longus, extensor hallucis longus, flexor digitorum longus, flexor hallucis longus, tibialis anterior muscles) | |
| **V**<br>One main and multiple secondary vascular pedicles<br>(pectoralis major, latissimus dorsi muscles) | |

# SKIN AND SOFT TISSUE SURGERY

## TNM classification of skin carcinoma
(except eyelid, penis, vulva)
T1 ≤ 2 cm
T2 ≤ 5 cm
T3 > 5 cm
T4  Infiltration of deeper extradermal structures (cartilage, bone, skeletal muscle)
N1  Regional lymph node metastases

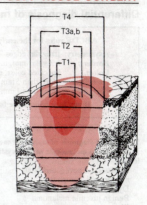

**Clark:** Clark's classification is by the level of tumor growth from the epidermis through the dermis (I–V).
*Clark's levels*:
I – contrast to epidermis and appendages
II – extension into papillary dermis
III – throughout papillary dermis impinging on reticular dermis
IV – invasion of reticular dermis
V – into subcutaneous fat
The treatment is determined by the thickness of the tumor and the presence of distant metastasis.
Breslow: *according to Breslow, extended exophytic growth worsens the prognosis*. Breslow classification measures maximum histologic thickness of tumor.

| Classification | | |
|---|---|---|
| Breslow | Clark | TNM |
| Melanoma *in situ* | I | Tis |
| ≤0.75 mm and/or infiltration of the papillary dermolayer | II | T1 |
| ≤1.5 mm and/or infiltration of the papillary layer | III | T2 |
| ≤3.0 mm and/or infiltration of the reticular layer | IV | T3a |
| ≤4.0 mm and/or infiltration of the reticular layer | IV | T3b |
| >4 mm and/or infiltration of the subcutis | V | T4a |
| Satellites within a 2 cm radius of the primary tumor | | T4b |
| Involvement of one or more lymph nodes 3 cm distant from primary | | N1 |
| Involvement of regional lymph nodes 3 cm distant from primary | | N2a |
| Cutaneous or subcutaneous satellites in the sphere of the regional lymph nodes more than 2 cm distant from the primary tumor | | N2b |
| N2a + N2b | | N2c |
| Distant metastases (cutis, subcutis, lymph nodes) | | M1a |
| Distant metastases (visceral) | | M1b |

# MEMORIX SURGERY

## Differential diagnosis of melanoma

> **ABCDE rules for the early recognition of 'malignant melanoma'**
>
> **Asymmetry:** Irregular edges
> **Borders:** Irregular margins
> **Color:** Speckled color, non-uniform pigmentation, light and dark
> **Diameter:** More than 5 mm
> **Elevation:** More than 1 mm
>
> **If any four criteria are fulfilled, suspect malignant melanoma**

**Differential diagnosis of malignant melanoma**

**1. Pigmented melanocyte or nevocystic lesions**
- Melanocytic nevi (junctional, intradermal, compound)
- Dysplastic nevus
- Benign juvenile melanoma
- Blue nevus
- Spitz nevus
- Lentigo maligna
- Halo nevus

**2. Epithelial lesions**
- Seborrhoic keratosis
- Melanoacanthoma
- Pigmented basal cell carcinoma
- Verruca vulgaris (common wart, hemorrhagic)
- Clear cell acanthoma
- Black hydrocystoma

**3. Vascular lesions**
- Hemangiopericytoma
- Granuloma pyogenicum
- Angiokeratoma
- Glomus tumor
- Subungual hemorrhage
- Kaposi's sarcoma

**4. Dermal lesions**
- Pigmented dermatofibroma
- Malignant fibrous histiocytoma
- Neurofibroma (rarely)

## Treatment

**Stages**

T1  Excision with 1–2-cm peripheral margins to a depth of the muscle fascia
T2  Excision with a 3-cm peripheral margin to a depth of the muscle fascia
T3+ Excision with a 3–5-cm peripheral margin and possible node dissection

Lymphadenectomy, adjuvant chemotherapy, and hyperthermic limb perfusion may be used in selected cases.

# SKIN AND SOFT TISSUE SURGERY

## Classification of soft tissue tumors

### Histologic classification of soft tissue tumors
(From Emzinger and Weiss (1988))

**I. Tumors and tumor-like lesions of fibrous tissue**

**Benign**
Fibroma
Elastofibroma
Fibroma of tendon sheath
Nuchal fibroma
Nasopharyngeal fibroma
Nodular fasciitis
Proliferative fasciitis
Proliferative myositis
Keloid

**Fibrous tumors of infancy and childhood**
Calcifying aponeurotic fibroma
Fibrous hamartoma
Fibromatosis
Hyalin fibromatosis
Fibromatosis of the neck
Myofibromatosis
Gingival fibromatosis
Giant cell fibroblastoma

**Superficial fibromatosis** (palmar and plantar, penile (Peytonie's), Kuncke pads)

**Deep fibromatosis** (intra-abdominal, extra-abdominal, mesenteric (Gardner's syndrome), postradiation, cicatricial)

**Malignant: fibrosarcoma** (adult, congenital, infantile, inflammatory, postradiation, cicatricial)

**II. Fibrohistiocytic tumors**

**Benign**
Fibrous histiocytoma
Atypical fibroxanthoma
Juvenile xanthogranuloma
Reticulohistiocytoma
Xanthoma

**Intermediate**
Dermatofibrosarcoma protuberans
Bednar tumor

**Malignant**
Fibrous histiocytoma
Storiform-pleomorphic
Myxofibrosarcoma
Giant cell tumor of soft parts
Inflammatory (malignant xanthogranuloma, xanthosarcoma)
Angiomatoid

**III. Tumors and tumor-like lesions of adipose tissue**

**Benign**
Lipoma
Angiolipoma
Spindle cell and pleomorphic lipoma
Lipoblastoma and lipoblastomatosis
Angiomyolipoma
Myelolipoma
Intramuscular and intermuscular lipoma
Lipoma of tendon sheath
Lumbosacral lipoma
Intraneural and perineural fibrolipoma
Diffuse lipomatosis
Cervical symmetrical lipomatosis (Madelung's disease)
Pelvic lipomatosis
Hibernoma

**Malignant: liposarcoma** (predominantly well differentiated: lipoma-like, sclerosing, imflammatory, myxoid, round cell, pleomorphic, dedifferentiated)

**IV. Tumors of muscle tissue**

**Smooth muscle**

**Benign**
Leiomyoma (cutaneous and deep)
Angiomyoma (vascular)
Epithelioid leiomyoma (benign leiomyoblastoma)
Intravenous leiomyomatosis
Leiomyomatosis peritonealis disseminata

**Malignant**
Leiomyosarcoma
Epithelioid leiomyosarcoma (malignant leiomyoblastoma)

**Striated muscle**

**Benign**
Adult rhabdomyoma
Genital rhabdomyoma
Fetal rhabdomyoma

**Malignant: rhabdomyosarcoma** (predominantly: embryonal, alveolar, pleomorphi, ectomesenchymoma (rhabdomyosarcoma with ganglion cell differentiation)

**V. Tumors and tumor-like lesions of blood vessels**

**Benign**
Hemangioma (capillary, cavernous, arteriovenous, venous, epithelioid (angiolymphoid hyperplasia, Kimura's disease), granulation tissue type (pyogenic granuloma))

**Deep hemangioma (intramuscular, synovial, perineural)**
Hemangiomatosis
Glomus tumor
Hemangiopericytoma
Papillary endothelial hyperplasia (intravascular vegetans hemangioendothelioma of Masson)

**Intermediate**
Hemangioendothelioma (epithelioid, spindle cell, malignant endovascular papillary angioendothelioma)

**Malignant**
Angiosarcoma
Kaposi's sarcoma
Malignant glomus tumor
Malignant hemangiopericytoma

# MEMORIX SURGERY

**VI. Tumors of lymph vessels**
 **Benign**
  Lymphangioma (cavernous, cystic hygroma)
  Lymphangiomatosis
  Lymphangiomyoma and lymphangiomyomatosis

 **Malignant**
  Angiosarcoma

**VII. Tumors and tumor-like lesions of synovial tissue**
 **Benign**
  Giant cell tumor of tendon sheath (localized nodular tenosynovitis, diffuse florid synovitis)

 **Malignant**
  Synovial sarcoma malignant synovioma (predominantly biphasic fibrous and epithelial, monophasic fibrous or epithelial, malignant giant cell tumor of tendon sheath)

**VIII. Tumors of mesothelial tissue**
 **Benign**
  Localized fibrous mesothelioma (subserosal fibroma)
  Multicystic peritoneal mesothelioma
  Exothelioma of the genital tract (adenomatoid tumor)

 **Malignant**
  Diffuse and localized mesothelioma (predominantly epithelial, fibrous, biphasic)

**IX. Tumors and tumor-like lesions of peripheral nerves**
 **Benign**
  Traumatic neuroma
  Morton's neuroma
  Neuromuscular hamartoma
  Nerve sheath ganglion
  Neurilemoma (benign schwannoma)
  Solitary neurofibroma (localized, diffuse, Pacinian, pigmented)
  Granular cell tumor
  Neurofibromatosis (von Recklinghausen's disease) (localized, plexiform, diffuse)
  Pigmented neuroectodermal tumor of infancy
  Ectopic meningioma
  Nasal glioma
  Neurothekoma

 **Malignant**
  Malignant schwannoma (including malignant schwannoma with rhabdomyoblastic differentiation (malignant Triton tumor), glandular malignant schwannoma, and epithelioid malignant schwannoma)
  Peripheral tumors of primitive neuroectodermal tissues
  Malignant pigmented neuroectodermal tumor of infancy
  Malignant granular cell tumor

**X. Tumors of autonomic ganglia**
 **Benign**
  Ganglioneuroma
  Melanocytic schwannoma

 **Malignant**
  Neuroblastoma
  Ganglioneuroblastoma
  Malignant melanocytic schwannoma

**XI. Tumors of paraganglionic structures**
 **Benign**
  Paraganglioma (solitary, multiple, familial)

 **Malignant**
  Malignant paraganglioma

**XII. Tumors and tumor-like lesions of cartilage and bone-forming tissues**
 **Benign**
  Panniculitis ossificans
  Myositis ossificans
  Fibrodysplasia (myositis) ossificans progressiva
  Extraskeletal chondroma or osteochondroma
  Extraskeletal osteoma

 **Malignant**
  Extraskeletal chondrosarcoma (well differentiated, myxoid (chordoid sarcoma), mesenchymal, extraskeletal osteosarcoma

**XIII. Tumors and tumor-like lesions of pluripotential mesenchyme**
 **Benign**
  Congenital granular cell tumor
  Tumoral calcinosis
  Myxoma (cutaneous and intramuscular)
  Aggressive angiomyxoma
  Amyloid tumor
  Parachroma
  Mesenchymoma

 **Malignant**
  Alveolar soft part sarcoma
  Epithelioid sarcoma
  Clear cell sarcoma of tendons and aponeuroses (malignant melanoma, soft parts)
  Extraskeletal Ewing's sarcoma
  Mesenchymoma

**XIV. Tumors and tumor-like lesions of disputed or uncertain origin**
  Histogenic
  Benign

**XV. Unclassified soft tissue tumors and tumor-like lesions**

## SKIN AND SOFT TISSUE SURGERY

## Treatment of soft tissue tumors
**Differential diagnosis between benign and malignant soft tissue tumors is difficult, consequently:**

> *Every soft tissue tumor*
> *requires early excisional biopsy*

**Principles of sarcoma resection**
Plan for a wide field of excision
(The tumor should not be visible to the surgeon during surgery)
Minimal manipulation of the tumor
Early central vein ligature to avoid hematogenous spread
Complete removal of the tumor capsule and the pseudo-capsule containing the growth, together with a wide margin of healthy tissue (muscle group resection or excision)
The fundamental principle is to obtain complete excision

**Characteristics of malignant soft tissue tumors**

Local recurrence common
Hematogenous metastasis to the lung lymphatic metastasis rare, rarely to the liver or other organs
Prognosis dependent on:
   size of tumor
   location of tumor
   tumor histology
Local recurrences are frequently due to incomplete primary excision

## MEMORIX SURGERY

## Classification of soft tissue sarcomas

**Adult**

T1 ≤ 5 cm
T2 > 5 cm

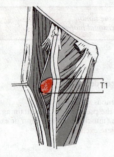
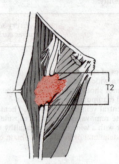

(T3 – Invasion of bones, large vessels or large nerves – the TNM classification is used to determine the extent of surgical resection and/or adjuvant therapy.)

# SKIN AND SOFT TISSUE SURGERY

## Wounds and wound healing: defects of skin and/or mucosa

| Wound types | Trauma |
|---|---|
| Cut, stab wounds | Sharp, pointed |
| Tear, crush wounds, contusions | Blunt |
| Tears, abrasions | Shearing |
| Combined injuries | |

**Stages of wound healing:** 1. Exudation (1–5 days); 2. Proliferation (6–21 days); 3. Remodeling (>21 days)

### Primary repair
Minimal scar formation
Primary suture of an elective surgical incision or a surgically débrided traumatic wound:

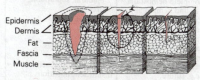

### Secondary wound healing
Defect forms granulation tissue and heals by contracture and epithelialization.

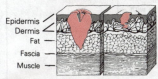

### Basics of wound care:
1. Cleansing of wound edges
   Leave open doubtful wounds (i.e. human bite)
   More caudally placed wounds (e.g. buttock, thigh and lower leg/foot) may be more difficult to obtain primary healing
2. Surgical débridement and irrigation to remove all foreign bodies and non-viable tissue
3. Careful handling of tissues
4. Atraumatic suture placement

Most common *Staphylococcal* infection

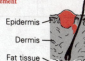

Acne  Folliculitis  Furuncle  Carbuncle

**Abscess:** operative drainage indicated
**Boil:** primary conservative treatment indicated

# MEMORIX SURGERY

## Clinical signs of acute inflammation

Calor (Heat)
Dolor (Pain)
Rubor (Redness)
Tumor (Swelling)
Impairment of function

## Disorders of wound healing

| Preoperative factors | Intraoperative factors | Postoperative factors |
|---|---|---|
| Obesity<br>Agranulocytosis<br>Alcoholism<br>Old age<br>  ($\downarrow$ fibroblast growth)<br>  ($\downarrow$ collagen formation)<br>Anemia<br>Diabetes mellitus<br>Hypogamma-<br>  globulinemia<br>Hypovolemia<br>Infection, sepsis<br>  (e.g. HIV infection)<br>Long preoperative<br>  hospitalization<br>Malignancy (e.g.<br>  leukemia, lymphoma)<br>Malnutrition (e.g.<br>  albumin, mineral,<br>  vitamin deficiency)<br>Medication (e.g.<br>  antipyretics, acetyl-<br>  salicylic acid,<br>  glucocorticoids,<br>  cytotoxics)<br>Renal failure<br>Cirrhosis of liver<br>Coagulopathies<br>Terminal disease<br>Neuropathies<br>Connective tissue disease | Tissue dehydration<br>  (long operative<br>  duration, deficient<br>  tissue hydration)<br>Incomplete hemostasis<br>  (wound hematoma)<br>Excessive electro-<br>  cauterization<br>  (necrosis)<br>Excessive suture<br>  material<br>Foreign-body reaction<br>  (e.g. suture<br>  granuloma, implant<br>  incompatibility)<br>Deficient hygiene<br>  (contamination with<br>  pathogenic<br>  organisms)<br>Inadequate blood flow<br>  in the sutured layer<br>Suture under tension<br>Residual cavities<br>  (seroma)<br>Crushing of wound<br>  edges (e.g. with<br>  forceps) | Long retention of catheter<br>  (endotracheal,<br>  gastroduodenal,<br>  intra-arterial, intravenous,<br>  epidural, suprapubic,<br>  urethral)<br>Inadequate:<br>  hygiene,<br>  patient care,<br>  dressing changes<br>Keloid formation<br>  ($\uparrow$ fibroblast reaction)<br>Insufficient nutrition |

# SKIN AND SOFT TISSUE SURGERY

## Tetanus

### Staging classification of tetanus infection
I    Muscular rigidity, opisthotonus, difficulty in swallowing, trismus
II   Compensated dyspnea, moderate liability to convulsions, strong muscular rigidity
III  Decompensated dyspnea, respiratory failure (intubation need), generalized cramp, fever, circulatory instability. Intensive care and muscle relaxants necessary

### Prophylaxis

| **Essential for** – all wounds<br>– **manipulating an old wound**<br>(e.g. surgical revision of an old war injury) |
|---|

| **Particularly dangerous wounds** | – deep and/or dirty wounds, particularly with foreign-body penetration, injuries with much tissue damage and reduced oxygen supply<br>– severe burns<br>– septic abortion<br>– tissue necrosis |
|---|---|

| **Prophylaxis in injury** | – surgical wound care (débridement)<br>– inoculation | |
|---|---|---|
| Inoculation status (number of prior immunizations) | All wounds | Additional, apart from clean, trivid wounds |
| unknown, 0–1 | T or Td* | TIG |
| 2 | T or Td* | TIG, if the injury is over 24 hours old |
| ≥3 | T or Td* if the last inoculation was more than 5 years previous (in clean insignificant wounds: ≥10 y.) | No TIG |
| *in children under 7y: DT instead of Td<br>T Tetanus toxoid (≥40 IU)<br>Td Tetanus–diphtheria toxoids (≥40 IU/≥4 IU)<br>DT Diphtheria–tetanus toxoids (≥30 IU/≥40 IU)<br>TIG Human tetanus–immunoglobulin | | |

### Basic immunization
– Initial: age 2, 4, 6, 18 months
– Three-injection tetanus inoculation or four-injection mixed inoculation (tetanus, diphtheria, pertussis)
– The interval between the inoculations should be at least 4 weeks

**Administration method – Intramuscular**

## Gas-forming wound infections: differential diagnosis

|  | *Clostridium* myonecrosis | *Clostridium* cellulitis | Streptococcal myositis | Infected vascular gangrene |
|---|---|---|---|---|
| Incubation | Less than 3 days | 3 days | 3–4 days | Over 5 days |
| Onset | Acute | Gradual | Subacute or insidious, lingering | Gradual |
| Toxemia | Extremely severe | Absent or slight | Severe after some time | Absent or light |
| Pain | Severe | Absent | Variable, mostly severe | Variable |
| Swelling | Marked | Absent or slight | Marked | Often doubtful |
| Skin | Tense, often conspicuously white | Little change | Tense, often copper-colored | Discolored, often black, with raised vesicles |
| Discharge | Variable – can be massive, serous–blood color (like cranberry juice) | Little or none | Copious or sero-purulent | None |
| Gas | Rare, unless terminal | Very copious | Very little | Very copious |
| Odor | Varied, often sweet | Putrid | Slight, occasionally acid | Putrid |
| Muscles | Massive changes | Not affected | Massive changes | Necrotic |

(After MacLennan (1962))

# SKIN AND SOFT TISSUE SURGERY

## Decubitus ulcers
### Predilection sites

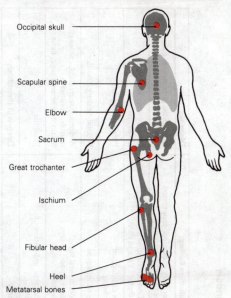

- Occipital skull
- Scapular spine
- Elbow
- Sacrum
- Great trochanter
- Ischium
- Fibular head
- Heel
- Metatarsal bones

### Daniel classification of decubitus ulcers
- **I** Skin redness
- **II** Superficial skin ulceration
- **III** Necrosis into the subdermal fat
- **IV** Necrosis into all deeper adjacent soft tissues
- **V** Extensive necrosis with osteitis, bony sequestration or joint destruction

### Seiler classification of wound condition
- **A** Wound 'clean', granulation tissue, no necrosis
- **B** Wound surface dirty, 'draining', residual necroses, no infiltration of underlying tissues
- **C** Wound as in stage B, with infiltration of underlying tissues and/or general infection (sepsis)

Both classifications may be combined, e.g. stage IIIB for a weeping decubitus ulcer with spread into the subdermal fat.

**Caution:** factors which place a patient at risk include prolonged immobilization, coma, debilitation, poor nutritional status and paraplegic neuropathy. Inadequate prophylaxis by medical personnel may lead to legal claims against the physician.

## Postoperative fever: differential diagnosis

### Evaluation of postoperative fever

| Patient's complaints | Physical examination findings | Diagnosis |
|---|---|---|
| Chest pain | Reduced respiratory excursion, suppressed respiration, weak breath sounds | Bronchitis, pneumonia, pulmonary embolism effusion, empyema |
| Burning on micturition Frequency, urgency | Transurethral catheterization? Indwelling catheter? Pain in flank? | Urinary tract infection Urosepsis |
| Pain in intravenous/arterial puncture site | Classical signs of infection Indwelling catheter | Phlebitis, sepsis |
| Pain in the surgical wound | Classical signs of infection | Wound-healing disorder |
| Abdominal pain | Sonography, peritoneal signs? Serum amylase + lipase, X-rays Abdominal sounds | Abscess, pancreatitis, cholangitis, sutures, peritonitis Secondary hemorrhage, ileus |
| Superficial pain in legs | Redness, tenderness, induration of superficial veins | Phlebitis |
| Severe leg pain | Deep tenderness | Deep-vein thrombosis |
| Earache | Tenderness, redness and protrusion of ear drum | Otitis media |
| Oral discomfort | Redness of mouth and trachea, white patches | *Candida* infection |
| Discomfort at site of drain | Redness at the tube perforation site | Wound infection, intra-abdominal abscess, empyema |
| **Allergic reaction** (medication, transfusion), medication-induced, tumor decay, malignancy (e.g. Hodgkin's disease, hypernephroma, leukemia), absorption from extended operation, trauma, collagenosis. | | |

# SKIN AND SOFT TISSUE SURGERY

## Fever of undetermined origin

**Definition:** an illness lasting at least 2 weeks with repeated peaks of temperature over 38.3°C and resistant to diagnosis after 1 week of intensive investigation

### Causes

After Jacoby and Swartz (1973)

### Infections
*Systemic*
- Miliary tuberculosis, tuberculosis
- Endocarditis (subacute bacterial)
- Rare infectious diseases: cytomegalovirus, toxoplasmosis, brucellosis, psittacosis, gonococcemia, meningococcal infection, disseminated mycosis, histoplasmosis, actinomycosis, malaria, listeriosis, infectious mononucleosis, AIDS

*Local*
- Liver: abscess, cholangitis
- Other visceral locations: pancreatitis, tubo-ovarian abscess, cholecystitis, empyema of gallbladder, silent perforation
- Intraperitoneal: subhepatic, subphrenic, paracolic, pelvic or retroperitoneal abscess, silent appendiceal perforation, interloop abscess, retrosigmoid abscess
- Urogenital: pyelonephritis, renal abscess, prostatic abscess

### Neoplasia (20%)
- Localized malignancy: lung, liver, kidney, pancreas, atrial myxoma
- Metastatic malignancy: melanoma, lung, kidney, gastrointestinal tract
- Reticuloendothelial: Hodgkin's disease, non-Hodgkin lymphoma, leukemia, multiple myeloma

### Collagen diseases (15%)
- Rheumatic fever, chronic polyarthritis, giant cell arteritis, lupus erythematosus

### Rarer causes
- Granulomatous: sarcoidosis, granulomatous hepatitis, specific granulomatous diseases
- Inflammatory bowel diseases: Crohn's disease, ulcerative colitis, granulomatous colitis
- Pulmonary embolism
- Medication fever
- Psychogenic: habitual hyperthermia, artificially induced (factitious) fever
- Cirrhosis of liver with active hepatocellular necrosis
- Various rare diseases (familial Mediterranean fever, Whipple's disease, Fabry's disease)
- Remaining undiagnosed 5–8%

### Diagnosis
- History (especially occupation, distant foreign travel, epidemiologic considerations)
- Physical examination (cardiovascular, lungs, gastrointestinal, urogenital)
- Immunologic, microbial, serologic investigations
- Cytologic, histologic investigation of body fluids or tissues and other microbiologic examinations (e.g. fine-needle biopsy)
- Gallium scan, indicum scan, CT scan
- Frequent review of history and physical exam

## MEMORIX SURGERY

# HIV infection/AIDS

**HIV** – human immunodeficiency virus
**AIDS** – acquired immunodeficiency syndrome

**At-risk groups**

Medical and surgical personnel should take the necessary precautions when treating the acute or chronically ill patient who is:
- male bi- or homosexual
- intravenous drug user
- hemophiliac
- a recipient of blood or plasma transfusion

Remember that any person is potentially infected. Always use universal precautions to avoid exposure to blood and body fluids.

**Transmission pathways**
- Blood, blood components, body fluids
- Sexual practices
- Injection needles, scalpels, surgical needles, pointed instruments
- Placental, perinatal
- Transfusion (plasma, blood, blood components)
- Transplantation (organ transplants)

**Classification of HIV diseases [Centers for Disease Control (CDC)]**

**I** Acute HIV infection

**II** Asymptomatic HIV infection

**III** Lymphadenopathic syndrome (LAS)
Persistent generalized lymphadenopathy (PGL)

**IV** A – nonspecific symptoms (fever >30 days, weight loss >10%, diarrhea >30 days)

B – neurological diseases (dementia, myelopathy, peripheral neuropathy)

C – 1. Opportunistic infection
2. Other infection (candidiasis, tuberculosis, recurrent salmonellosis, oral leukoplakia)

D – secondary neoplasia

E – other diseases (lymphoma, interstitial pneumonia)

TB, cervical cancer added in 1993 as was $CD_4 < 200$ by itself.

# SKIN AND SOFT TISSUE SURGERY

**Special considerations during surgical intervention**

- The particular procedure must take into consideration not only the situation of the patient, but also the safety of the operative team and that of the postoperative attending medical personnel
- Restrict the indications for elective operations (? HIV testing)
- Consider the possibility of incomplete wound healing (e.g. in anorectal procedures)
- Consider the specific morbidity, mortality and life expectation
- Choose the technically easier and less traumatic operative method if there is an alternative procedure

**Prophylaxis**

- Safeguard against contamination and injury
- Wear gloves if contacting body fluids or mucous membranes; frequent changing of gloves if permeability is suspected
- Wear facemasks and protective spectacles to guard against aerosol contamination
- Wear double gloves and waterproof clothing during the operation
- The operation is performed by an experienced operative team used to working together
- Special operative technique:

    An open-minded and clear choice of operation

    Caution against injury from sharp incision retractors

    Use diathermy or laser coagulation in preference to understitching

    Insert sutures using needle holders instead of hand-held needles

    If there is an alternative operative method, choose the technically easier method
- Immediate and thorough attention to contaminated needles and sharp instruments, such as scalpels, after use
- Staff to refrain from invasive procedure and subsequent postoperative care of the patient if they have injuries or inflammation of skin
- Secure safe decontamination throughout case

**Procedure to follow if contaminated with HIV-positive material from needles, scalpels, etc.**

- Immediate cessation of surgical activity
- Intensive disinfection with bleeding injuries
- Institute the usual recognized medical routine procedures
- HIV testing of patient (with his permission)
- HIV testing of the injured person immediately, and after 42, 84, 180 and 365 days
- Administer zidovudine (AZT, ZdV) 200 mg 5 times a day for 42 days (the literature gives varying opinions of the value of AZT)

# MEMORIX SURGERY

## Facial fractures

### Important signs and symptoms

#### Most important symptoms

1 Malocclusion – could represent mandible, maxillary or alveolar fracture
2 Cheek and upper lip numbness – due to compression or laceration of the infraorbital nerve – ($V^2$), may represent zygoma tripod fracture
3 Diplopia – double vision – may represent orbital floor fracture with entrapment of extraocular muscles
4 Nasal bleeding – nasal bone fracture
5 Tinnitus – basilar skull fracture

#### Important physical signs

1 Mobile maxilla – LeFort fractures
2 Traumatic telecanthus – separation of medial canthi. Suggests naso-orbital ethmoid fracture
3 Trismus – painful opening of jaws, mandibular fracture, condylar fracture
4 Orbital hematoma – (raccoon's eyes), maxillary orbital or basilar skull fracture
5 Battle's sign – hematoma over mastoid process – suggests basilar skull fracture
6 Anterior open bite – suggests alveolar fracture, bilateral temporomandibular joint dislocation, bilateral condylar fractures of mandible, central midface (LeFort fractures)
7 Lateral open bite – unilateral LeFort fracture, unilateral temporomandibular joint dislocation or condylar fracture

### Diagnosis

- The most important tool in diagnosis of facial fractures is the physical examination
- Plain facial X-rays, panorex X-ray for mandible, Townes view for condyles of mandible
- Prone coronal or axial CT scan for orbital floors (3-mm cuts)

### LeFort fractures

I    Horizontal fracture of maxillary alveolar process
II   Pyramidal fracture of maxilla
III  Transverse facial fracture through the orbits (cranial facial dysfunction)

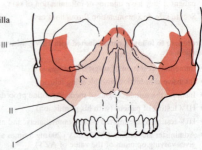

# Lymphoma in neck region
## Scheme for diagnosis of lymphomas in the neck region
(From Zuhlke and Hals (1990))

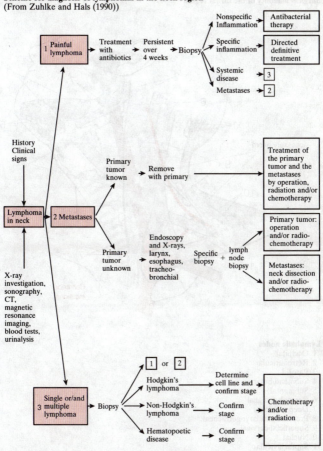

## MEMORIX SURGERY

# Lymphoma in throat region

**Surgical anatomy of the throat region**

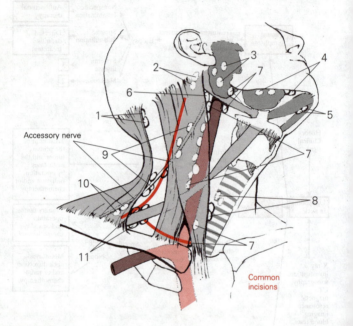

Accessory nerve

Common incisions

**Lymphatic nodes**
1. Occipital
2. Retroauricular
3. Parotid
4. Submandibular
5. Submental
6. Retropharyngeal
7. Deep cervical
8. Pre- and paralaryngotracheal
9. Superficial cervical
10. Nuchal
11. Supraclavicular

**Caution:** division of the accessory nerve is a frequent surgical malpractice.

## SURGERY OF THE FACE AND NECK

# Lateral and median throat tumors

**Differential diagnosis**
(After Zühlke H., 1990)

**Lateral**

Lymphoma (specific and nonspecific inflammation)
Systemic disease, metastasis
Branchial cleft cyst or sinus

Neurogenic tumor
Vascular tumor
Parotid tumor

Laryngocele
Congenital cyst
Thyroid tumor

Mesenchymal tumor
Lymphoma

Teratoma
Vascular tumor
Lymphangioma

**Median**

Submental lymphoma
Desmoid
Ectopic salivary gland tissue

Median cyst
Ectopic thyroid tissue (thyroglossal duct cyst)
Thyroid tumor

Ectopic thymus tissue

Desmoid
Lymphoma

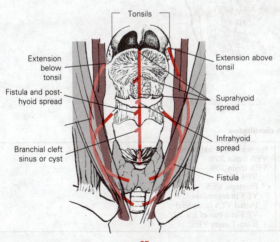

# ECG/LOWN classification

**ECG – Extremity leads**
right arm: red
left arm: yellow
left leg: green
right leg: black (earth)

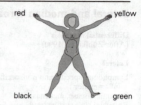

**ECG – Chest wall leads (unipolar, Wilson)**
$V_{1-4}$ ICR (intercostal space) right parasternal
$V_{2-4}$ ICR left parasternal
$V_3$ – between $V_2$ and $V_4$
$V_{4-5}$ ICR in the mediocclavicular line
$V_5$ – at top of $V_4$, in the left anterior axillary line
$V_6$ – at top of $V_4$, in the left median axillary line

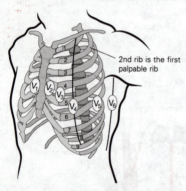

2nd rib is the first palpable rib

ECG chest wall leads

## LOWN classification

| | |
|---|---|
| 0 | No ventricular extrasystoles (VES) |
| 1a | VES 1/min 30/h |
| 1b | VES 1/min 30/h |
| 2 | VES 30/h |
| 3a | Polytope VES |
| 3b | VES in bigeminus |
| 4a | Paired VES (couplets) |
| 4b | VES in a run of ES >3 |
| 5 | R-on-T early VES |

# HEART AND THORAX SURGERY

## Congenital heart defects

Congenital heart defects – including malformations of the great vessels – occur in around 1% (0.8–1.2%) of all newborns

| Frequency of congenital heart defects | (%) |
|---|---|
| Patent ductus arteriosus | 10 |
| Aortic isthmus stenosis (coarctation) | 5 |
| Thoracic vessel anomalies (rings, loops) | 1.2 |
| Aortic stenosis | 7 |
| Pulmonary stenosis | 10 |
| Atrial septal defects | 10 |
| Ventricular septal defects | 28 |
| Complete A–V canal defects | 2 |
| Total anomalous pulmonary venous drainage | 1.4 |
| Common truncus arteriosus | 1.5 |
| Tetralogy of Fallot | 10 |
| Transposition of the great arteries | 5 |
| Ebsteinanomaly of the tricuspid valve | 0.3 |
| Tricuspid atresia | 1.2 |
| Univentricular heart | 1.5 |
| Coronary artery anomalies | 0.3 |

From Keith *et al.* (1978)

| Acyanotic group without shunt | Frequency | |
|---|---|---|
| Isolated pulmonary stenosis | 10% | – Valvular<br>– Infundibular |
| Isolated aortic stenosis | 7% | – Valvular<br>– Subvalvular<br>– Supravalvular |
| Aortic isthmus stenosis | 5% | |

**Aortic stenoses**
I   Supravalvular
II  Valvular
III Subvalvular

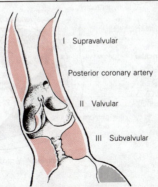

I Supravalvular

Posterior coronary artery

II Valvular

III Subvalvular

## MEMORIX SURGERY

**Acyanotic group with shunt – frequency**
(left-right-short-circuit connection)

| | |
|---|---|
| Atrial septum defect | |
| primum or secundum type | 10% |
| Ventricular septal defect (VS) | 28% |
| Complete A–V canal | 2% |
| Patent ductus arteriosus | 10% |
| Aortopulmonary window | |
| Rare types | |

**The most common defect is ventricular septal (VS) defect at 28%**

**Caution:** watch out for the development of fixed pulmonary hypertension and shunt reversal with cyanosis

**Reversal syndrome** – in the newborn and hemodynamically significant shunt

**Treatment**
Closure of a hemodynamically significant ventricular septal defect in the first weeks and months of life until 1 year of age

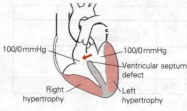

**Localization of ventricular septum (VS) defects**
I arterial (conal)
II perimembranous
III atrioventricular (A–V) canal type
IV muscular type

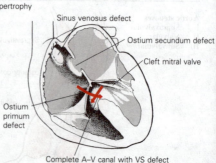

# HEART AND THORAX SURGERY

**Cyanotic group with shunt (right–left)**

| Tetralogy of Fallot (10%) | Ventricular septal defect, valvular or infundibular pulmonary stenosis, dextroposition of the aorta, right ventricular hypertrophy |
|---|---|
| Transposition of the great vessels (5%) | Aorta from the right ventricle |
| Truncus arteriosus (1.4%) | Common trunk for aorta and pulmonary artery |
| Univentricular heart | |

**Tetralogy of Fallot**

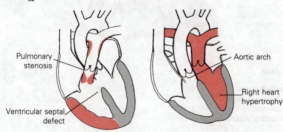

Pulmonary stenosis
Ventricular septal defect
Aortic arch
Right heart hypertrophy

**Treatment**

| Tetralogy of Fallot | **Palliative operation** in the first month of life<br>**Blalock–Taussig shunt:** anastomosis between the subclavian and pulmonary arteries<br>**Waterston:** aortopulmonary anastomosis<br>**Brock:** resection of the infundibular stenosis<br>**Total correction:** closure of the ventricular septum defect, valvulotomy of the pulmonary valve, resection of the infundibular stenosis |
|---|---|
| **Transposition of the great vessels (TGA)** | Survival only possible with an auricular defect, ventricular septum defect or patent ductus arteriosus<br>**Treatment of choice:** creation of an auricular septum defect in the first hours of life – balloon septostomy (Raschkind) or septum resection – Blalock–Hanlon<br>**Total correction:** anatomic resection within the first 10 days of life or auricular reversal (Senning, Mustard) within the first 12 months |
| **Truncus arteriosus** | **Correction of the truncus arteriosus:** connect the right ventricle to the pulmonary artery |
| **Univentricular heart** | Fontan operation |

## MEMORIX SURGERY

## Congenital deformities of the great vessels

### Patent ductus arteriosus (10%)

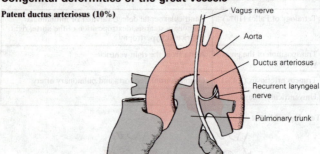

Left–right shunt

**Dangers in prematures**
Pulmonary hypertension
Bacterial endocarditis
Dyspnea requiring urgent operation

**Operation**
Ligature and suture or division and oversewing the stumps
Mortality <1%

**Aortic isthmus stenosis (5%)**
(*coarctation of the aorta*)
Coarctation is frequently associated with other deformities, above all patent ductus arteriosus

**Ventricular septum defect**
Aortic valve stenosis
Transposition of the great vessels

**Main symptoms:**
Brachiocephalic pressure rise
Loss of pulse in lower extremities

**Urgent operation:** for dyspnea in infancy

**Operative technique:**
Resection of the stenosis and end-to-end anastomosis in children and adults
Direct and indirect patch angioplasty (widening-patch)
Waldhausen's angioplasty operation in infants
Prosthesis interposition in adults
Mortality (all operative techniques) around 5%

# HEART AND THORAX SURGERY

## Acquired heart defects

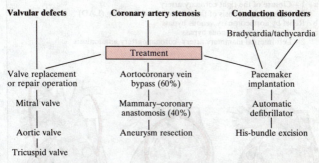

Operations for diseases of the coronary vascular system are performed in 500–1000 per million people worldwide (operative mortality 1–3%).

## Coronary arteries

(International Nomenclature Commission, Leningrad (1970), after Kaltenbach and Roskamm (1980))

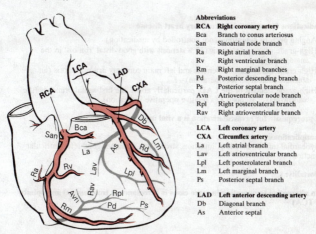

**Abbreviations**

| | |
|---|---|
| **RCA** | **Right coronary artery** |
| Bca | Branch to conus arteriosus |
| San | Sinoatrial node branch |
| Ra | Right atrial branch |
| Rv | Right ventricular branch |
| Rm | Right marginal branches |
| Pd | Posterior descending branch |
| Ps | Posterior septal branch |
| Avn | Atrioventricular node branch |
| Rpl | Right posterolateral branch |
| Rav | Right atrioventricular branch |
| **LCA** | **Left coronary artery** |
| **CXA** | **Circumflex artery** |
| La | Left atrial branch |
| Lav | Left atrioventricular branch |
| Lpl | Left posterolateral branch |
| Lm | Left marginal branch |
| Ps | Posterior septal branch |
| **LAD** | **Left anterior descending artery** |
| Db | Diagonal branch |
| As | Anterior septal |

## Coronary surgery

a  1 – Closure of the right coronary artery
   2 – High-grade stenosis of the left anterior descending (LAD)
b  Relief by aortocoronary venous bypass
c  1 – Aortocoronary venous bypass
   2 – Left internal mammary artery–coronary artery anastomosis

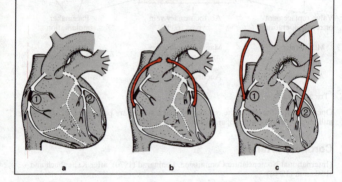

**Indications for operation in coronary heart disease**

Angina pectoris symptoms (not controlled by medication)
High-grade proximal stenosis (70% stenosis with good distal 'run-off' in the angiography)
High-grade multivascular stenosis and left main coronary artery stenosis (an absolute indication for operation)
High-grade stenosis of the LAD, particularly above the first septal branches (the 'widow-maker stenosis') (a relative operative indication)

**A prerequisite for revascularization is a vital myocardium.**

**Complications:**
Myocardial infarct, bleeding, infection, stroke, etc. (assumes good left ventricular function)

**Mortality:** 1%

**An alternative to operation in some cases is percutaneous transluminal angioplasty (PTCA)**

# HEART AND THORAX SURGERY

## Myocardial aneurysm

### Indications for operative treatment

Cardiac insufficiency (congestive heart failure)
Ventricular tachycardia
Distal vascular embolization
Coronary stenosis and angina

### Treatment

Resection of aneurysm with ventricle reconstruction and bypass of coronary stenosis, thrombectomy

Ablation of ectopic irritable foci in tachycardias by local cryosurgery or endocardial resection

Operative mortality: 5%

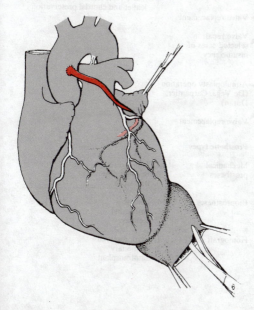

**Aneurysm resection and coronary artery bypass**

# *MEMORIX SURGERY*

## Acquired heart valve defects

### Heart valvular deficiencies

**Treatment**

**Mitral valve** → Stenosis →
- Stretching (Tubbs) rare
- Balloon valvuloplasty
- Open commissurotomy
- Valve replacement

→ Insufficiency →
- Valve repair, mitral annuloplasty with prosthetic valve ring (Carpentier, Duran *et al.*)
- Valve replacement (with or without leaflet and chordal preservation)

**Aortic valve** →
- Valve replacement
- Valve repair in selected cases of insufficiency

**Tricuspid valve** →
- Annuloplasty operation (De Vega, Carpentier, Duran)
- Valve replacement

### Prosthetic types

Mechanical prostheses
1. Tilting disc
2. Bileaflet disc
3. Ball-valve

Bioprostheses
1. Porcine
2. Pericardial
3. Stentless

Homograft
1. Cryopreserved
2. Pulmonary autotransplant

# HEART AND THORAX SURGERY

## Artificial heart valves

Auscultatory findings with different heart valves functioning normally

| | Ball-valve | Tilting disc type | Bileaflet valve | Bioprosthesis |
|---|---|---|---|---|
| Representative model | Starr–Edwards | Björk–Shiley, Medtronic Hall | St. Jude Medical | Xenograft, homograft or porcine graft |
| Related models | Harken, Cooley-Cutter, Smeloff-Cutter, McGovern, Braunwald-Cutter, De Bakey | Wada-Cutter, Lillehei-Kaster, Hall-Kaster, Omniscience, Medtronic | Carbomedics, Duromedics | Hancock, Angell-Shiley, Carpentier-Edwards, Microflow |
| Blood-flow pattern | | | | |

## Postoperative progress supervision

| History | Clinical examination | ECG | Mechanical cardiogram | Echo | X-rays | Laboratory |
|---|---|---|---|---|---|---|
| Subjective improvement | Auscultation findings | Rhythm | STI | Functioning of the prosthesis | Size of heart | Hemolysis |
| Effort capacity | Dyspnea | Signs of injury or hypertrophy as well as dysrhythmias | The ratio of the heart tones | Diameter of the cavities | Signs of congestion | |
| Complications | Crisp mechanical valve sound | | | LV function | Movement of the prosthesis | |
| | Ejection murmur | | | | Movement of the closure object | |

## HEART AND THORAX SURGERY

# Heart pacemaker

Bradycardiac disorders of rhythm
Stokes–Adams syndrome – acute
asystole with cerebral hypoxia after
temporary/permanent A–V block

**Operative access**
1. Cephalic vein
2. Subclavian vein
3. External jugular vein
4. Internal jugular vein

## Causes
- Coronary circulatory disorder
- Myocarditis
- Digitalis toxicity
  bradycardia

**Medication treatment**
**Sympathomimetics**
Operation: Pacemaker implantation

**Catheter electrode**
Combined sensor and stimulation electrodes

**Pacemaker**
- vertical pacing
- QRS triggered
- QRS inhibited
- atrial pacing

| VVI | Chamber stimulation as required  Chamber inhibited (triggered) |

| DDD | Atrial-paced  Ventricle not inhibited |

**Pacemaker batteries – Life 10–12 years**
Falling off in pacemaker's frequency indicates battery exhaustion

# MEMORIX SURGERY

**Tachycardiac heart rhythm disorders**

**Causes of sudden cardiac death**
- Coronary heart disease complicated by ventricular arrhythmia
- Continuous tachycardia with acquired valvular defects (CHF)
- Mitral valve prolapse
- Ventricular myocardial failure
- Myocardial infarction with cardiogenic failure

**Non-medical management of arrhythmias**
- anti-tachycardiac stimulation procedures by implanted rapid pacemaker system
- interception of A–V conduction by electro-shock (Bundle of His ablation)
- automatic cardioversion/defibrillation with implantable electro-shock apparatus

| Anti-arrhythmic cardiac surgery | Surgical procedure |
| --- | --- |
| **Sinus tachycardia**<br>Sinus node re-entry<br>Separation tachycardias | 1 Section of bundle of His<br>2 Sinus node isolation (excision, and re-implantation)<br>3 Maze procedure<br>   A–V node ablation and placement of pacemaker |
| **WPW**<br>(Wolff–Parkinson–White) syndrome<br>Accessory track (Kent bundle) | 1 Division of accessory pathways (Bundle of Kent)<br>2 Destruction by cryo or laser technique |
| Ventricular tachycardia | 1 Endocardial resection of irritable focus<br>2 Elimination by circumferential ventricular invasion<br>3 Elimination by cryosurgery<br>4 Aneurysm resection and excision with revascularization<br>5 Implantable defibrillator for 'poor ventricle' (EF < 20%)<br>6 Heart transplantation |

**Commonly used pacemakers**

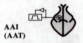

**AAI (AAT)**
Atrium paced as required, sensed and inhibited (triggered)

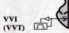

**VVI (VVT)**
Ventricle paced as required, sensed and inhibited (triggered)

**VAT**
Atrium sensed, ventricle paced. Pacing triggered

**DD**
Atrium sensed chamber paced as required

**DVI**
Sequential atrial and ventricular pacing required. Pacing inhibited

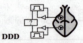

**DDD**
Dual chamber sensing and pacing. AV activity inhibits, atrial activity triggers pacing

## HEART AND THORAX SURGERY

# New York Heart Association (NYHA) classification

**Classification** of cardiac insufficiency or coronary heart disease (Criteria Committee, New York Heart Association (1964)).

| Class | Grading according to effort-dependent occurrence of symptoms: Dyspnea and/or angina pectoris or also exhaustion, palpitation, etc. |
|---|---|
| (0) | Asymptomatic |
| I | Severe effort without complaint (abnormal physical exertion can lead to symptoms) |
| II | Symptoms caused by raised, not unusual, effort; symptom-free on light effort |
| III | Symptoms on light effort; symptom-free at rest |
| IV | Symptoms at rest: no exertion possible |

**Therapeutic classification (after NHYA)**

A  No restriction of physical exercise necessary

B  Customary physical exercise need not be restricted, but abnormal, severe, or repeated effort should be restricted

C  Customary physical effort should be moderately restricted, and avoided if continuous

D  Normal physical effort should clearly be restricted

E  Patient should avoid exertion, at bed rest or in armchair

# Heart transplantation

**Indications for heart transplantation**
(International Society for Heart Transplantation, Official report, 1990)

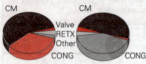

|  | Total | Youngest | Oldest |
|---|---|---|---|
| Heart |  |  |  |
| – orthotopic | 12319 | 1 day | 78 |
| – heterotopic | 312 | 3 months | 70 |
| Lungs |  |  |  |
| – heart and lung | 785 | 2 months | 60 |
| – 1 lung | 157 | 1 year | 63 |
| – both lungs | 48 | 14 years | 60 |

CM, cardiomyopathy;
CONG, congenital heart disease;
RETX, re-transplantation.

### Age limits

Age of subject (1 day to 78 years)
Age 44 years

### Indication for dilated cardiomyopathy (proportion of patients 50%)

Cardiac performance: NYHA III–IV
Ejection fraction: ≤20%
Biopsy: muscle fiber reduction
Increase in interstitial volume
Ventricular dysrhythmias (frequent)
Recurrent decompensation

### Indication in coronary heart disease (proportion of patients 41%)

Diffuse coronary artery disease not amenable to CABG
Cardiac wall aneurysm with minimal contractile portion
State after ineffective bypass operation and/or aneurysm resection
Operation for uncontrollable arrhythmias

### Rare indications

Heart valve disease (4%)
Re-transplantation
Treatment-resistant arrhythmias
Amyloidosis
Heart tumors

### Indication in children: 35% due to congenital cardiac defects

# HEART AND THORAX SURGERY

**Registry of the International Society for Heart Transplantation**

**Official Report**

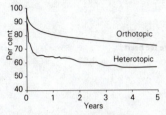

Survival rate of orthotopic and heterotopic heart transplants. Orthotopic transplants (70% after 5 years)

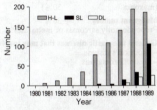

Number per year of heart–lung and lung transplants. H-L, heart–lung; SL, one lung; DL, both lungs

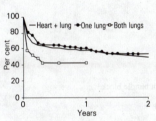

Survival rate after heart–lung and one or both lung tranplants

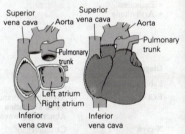

Operative field after removal of heart; atria (RA, LA) and great vessels remain

Operative field after complete heart transplant showing anastomoses of auricle and great vessels

### Selection criteria
- Age under 60–65 years
- No serious thoracic trauma
- No infection
- ABO compatibility
- Negative lymphocyte cross-match
- Adequate extrathoracic organ function (i.e. renal, hepatic)
- No active malignancy

# MEMORIX SURGERY

## Cardiac tumors

**Frequency:** 0.06% of all tumors

**Benign tumors**         70%
(myxoma                   30%)

**Malignant tumors**      30%
Preponderantly sarcomas or metastases

**General neoplastic diseases that may involve the heart**
– Hodgkin's disease
– Neurofibromatosis

### Symptoms

**Hemodynamic**
- Obstruction of the atrial ventricular valve, with syncope
- Obstruction of the pulmonary or venous system outflow
- Embolism
- Arrhythmia

### Diagnosis

| | |
|---|---|
| Laboratory tests: | Negative |
| ECG: | Arrhythmia, branch bundle block |
| | **Atrial fibrillation** |
| | Abnormal P-waves |
| **X-rays:** | Cardiomegaly |
| **Echocardiogram:** (two-dimensional) | Method of choice – demonstrates tumor |
| **Angiocardiography:** | Injection into the vena cava or pulmonary artery |
| **Computed tomography:** | Method of choice |

### Operative methods
- Excision of tumor
- Valve replacement
- Autotransplantation
- Automatic defibrillator
- Heart transplantation

# HEART AND THORAX SURGERY

## Heart–lung machine (extracorporeal circulation)

Prolonged circulatory disconnection during correction of congenital and acquired heart defects is only possible with the use of the heart–lung machine

**Principle:** There are two main components:
Oxygenator: artificial lung
Roller-pump and tube-hose system: artificial circulation

**Venous diversion** with blood taken from the right atrium or femoral vein and returned into the aorta or femoral artery

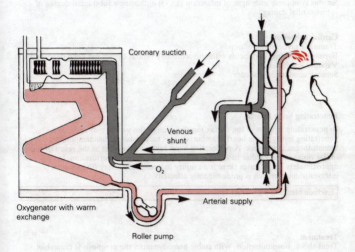

**Complications:**
Improper placement of cannula (from e.g. intima lesion, wall dissection, damage from neighboring structures)
Infection from contaminated, donated blood (HIV, hepatitis)
Air embolism during the injection into the atria or ventricles
Interruption of the blood source continuity
Peripheral thromboembolism
Increased tendency to bleeding due to the necessary heparinization and coagulopathy
Overdistention of the atrium and/or ventricle
Inadequate perfusion due to technical deficiency

# MEMORIX SURGERY

## Cardiac trauma

Up to 25% of all traffic injuries show a direct cardiac involvement

### Blunt cardiac injury predominates

Compression of the chest wall, i.e. from steering wheel
Sporting injuries
Occupational accidents

As a rule, symptoms are slight without evidence of ECG or enzyme changes

### Cardiac concussion
Serious symptoms with signs of infarction (ECG) indicating a substantial degree of myocardial damage

### Cardiac contusion
Traumatic myocardial infarction
Bypass thrombosis in patients with aortocoronary venous bypass has been described
Valvular insufficiency
Sensory conduction disorder

### Penetrating heart injuries

In penetrating injuries of the thorax the direction of the wound may indicate a penetrating injury of the heart chamber(s). This may cause cardiac tamponade, hematothorax, and shock. A perforating heart injury exists when as the result of the initial violence the cardiac function is affected by e.g. a bullet perforation. In approximately 5% of cases there is an injury to a coronary artery (the anterior interventricular branch is predominantly affected)

> **Exclude bleeding with heart tamponade**

### Treatment
Treat shock, hospitalization. With stable hemodynamics the prognosis is favorable: with unstable hemodynamics it is unfavorable.

Prognosis: 50–60% of patients with cardiac injuries due to gunshot wounds die immediately, but only 25% die from a stab injury

- The prognosis in ventricular and auricular injury is good, as the musculature often closes spontaneously and is sutureable

- Leave a penetrating object in place until in the operating room

- The diagnostic characteristic of cardiac tamponade: jugular venous distension, muffled heart tones, hypotension (Beck's triad)

- Pericardiocentesis

# HEART AND THORAX SURGERY

## Pericardial effusion/pericardiocentesis

### Symptoms

- Chest pain (marked in dry pericarditis)
- Dyspnea pain induced, restricted gaseous exchange
- Upper abdominal pain
- Dysphagia
- Faint heart sounds
- Drop in arterial pressure (narrow pulse pressure)
- Shock (tachycardia)
- Jugular venous distention
- Pulsus paradoxus

### Pericardial aspiration

- Approach between the xyphoid and the lower left rib border. Insert obliquely, at a 45° angle, the indwelling catheter can be left in place. The aspirating needle may be connected to an ECG lead. If the myocardium is contacted by the needle a pattern will be seen on the ECG.

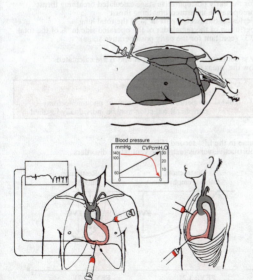

## MEMORIX SURGERY

## Preoperative assessment of lung function
(Modified from Konietzko *et al.* (1983))

**Basic diagnosis**
Spirometry (pre- and post-bronchodilator)
- overall estimation of the pulmonary functional state
- determination of any obstruction and restriction, instability of the respiratory passages

Lung perfusion scintigraphy with determination of 'areas of interest'
Arterial blood-gas analysis
Electrocardiography (ECG)

**Further examination** (directed to operative risk assessment)
Spiro-ergometry
Stress/ECG
Thallium cardiac scan
Coronary angiography
Whole-body plethysmography

**Estimation of postoperative expected** $FEV_1$ (forced expiration volume in 1 second)

$$FEV_1 \text{ postop.} = FEV_1 \text{ preop.} \times \frac{100 - A - K \times B}{100}$$

| | |
|---|---|
| $FEV_1$ postop. | – for the early postoperative stage calculated breathing thrust |
| $FEV_1$ preop. | – preoperative measured breathing thrust |
| A | – perfusion of resected part in % of the total lung |
| B | – perfusion of the remainder of the operated side in % of the total |
| K | – 0.37 (constant for the early postoperative stage) |

The preoperative FEV is confirmed spirometrically; A and B are calculated scintigraphically to show the 'areas of interest'

| $FEV_1$ postoperative | $\geq 2.5$ | no increase in operative risk |
|---|---|---|
| | $\leq 2.4$ | slightly raised risk |
| | 0.8–1.0 | inoperable for lobectomy or pneumonectomy peripheral resection may be individually justified |

**Tiffeneau's test**
Forced expiration volume in the first second ($FEV_1$)
for differentiation of obstructive versus restrictive ventilation disorders

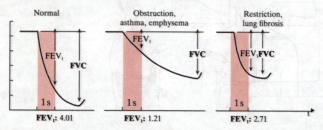

Normal — $FEV_1$: 4.01
Obstruction, asthma, emphysema — $FEV_1$: 1.21
Restriction, lung fibrosis — $FEV_1$: 2.71

# HEART AND THORAX SURGERY

## Bronchial tree: lobes, segments and lymph nodes

Segments 1–3: right upper lobe
Segments 4–5: right middle lobe
Segments 6–9: right lower lobe
Segments 1–5: left upper lobe
Segments 6–9: left lower lobe

**The bronchiopulmonary and tracheobronchial lymph nodes of the lung**

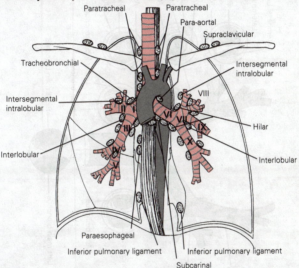

**Bronchial system with segment bronchi,**
**Right:**
I       right main bronchus
II      upper lobe stem bronchus
III     intermediate bronchus
IV      middle lobe right stem bronchus
V       lower lobe right stem bronchus

**Left:**
VI      left main bronchus
VII     upper lobe stem bronchus
VIII    stem of the apical segment
IX      stem of lingula
X       left lower lobe bronchus

**Regional lymph nodes**
- intrathoracic lymph nodes peribronchial: intersegmental, intralobar, interlobar, hila mediastinal: tracheobronchial, subcarinal, paratracheal, para-aortal, paraesophageal, pulmonary ligament, anterior mediastinum
- scalenus lymph nodes
- supraclavicular lymph nodes

## Bronchoscopic views

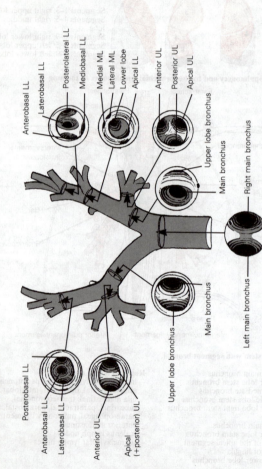

LL, lower lobe bronchus; ML, middle lobe bronchus; UL, upper lobe bronchus

# HEART AND THORAX SURGERY

## Lung lobes and segments

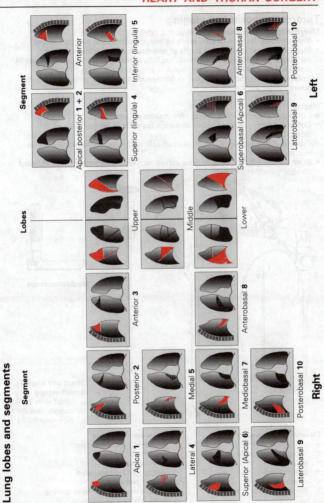

# Tumor diagnosis and staging

**Morphological confirmation** (histologic and cytologic differentiation)
- Bronchoscopy (suction biopsy, brush biopsy, transbronchial puncture biopsy)
- Mediastinoscopy (exclude N3 stages of non-small-cell bronchial carcinoma, peripheral areas of unclear diagnosis, exclude a small-cell bronchial carcinoma by computed tomography when lymphoma is present on staging)
- Transthoracic needle biopsy (only in functionally inoperable patients or when postoperative FEV is <0.8)

**Staging**
- Computed tomography of thorax (dimensions of tumor)
- Computed tomography of upper abdomen (to exclude liver or adrenal metastases)
- Computed tomography of skull (in small-cell carcinoma, on suspicion of brain metastasis)
- Bone scintigraphy (to exclude bone metastases) only with symptoms or elevated alkaline phosphatase level.

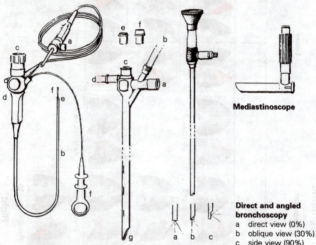

**Mediastinoscope**

**Direct and angled bronchoscopy**
a direct view (0%)
b oblique view (30%)
c side view (90%)

**Flexible bronchoscope**
a cold light attachment
b fiberglass light cable
c eyepiece
d control head
e objective
f flexible introducing forceps

**Injection bronchoscope**
a breathing tube attachment
b injection attachment
c viewing opening
d orifice for fiberglass cable
e rubber sleeve
f closure window with rapid opening
g bronchoscope lip

# Histologic classification of lung tumors (WHO, 1981)

I **Epithelial tumors**
  A Benign
    1 Papilloma
      a. Squamous epithelial papilloma
      b. Transitional cell papilloma
    2 Adenoma
      a. Pleomorphic adenoma
      b. Monomorphic adenoma
      c. Others
  B Dysplasia and carcinoma *in situ*
  C Malignant
    1 Squamous cell carcinoma
      a. Spindle cell carcinoma
    2 Small-cell carcinoma
      a. Oat cell carcinoma
      b. Intermediate cell type
      c. Combined oat cell carcinoma
    3 Adenocarcinoma
      a. Acinar adenocarcinoma
      b. Papillary adenocarcinoma
      c. Bronchoalveolar carcinoma
      d. Solid carcinoma with mucus formation
    4 Large-cell carcinoma
      a. Giant cell carcinoma
      b. Clear cell carcinoma
    5 Adenosquamous carcinoma
    6 Carcinoid
    7 Bronchial gland carcinoma
      a. Adenocystic carcinoma
      b. Mucoepidermal carcinoma
      c. Other
    8 Other carcinomas

II **Soft tissue tumors**

III **Mesothelial tumors**
  A Benign mesothelioma
  B Malignant mesothelioma
    1 Epithelial
    2 Fibrosing (spindle cell)
    3 Biphasic

IV **Different tumor types**
  A Benign
  B Malignant
    1 Carcinosarcoma
    2 Pulmonary blastoma
    3 Malignant melanoma
    4 Others

V **Secondary tumors**

VI **Unclassified tumors**

VII **Tumor-like lesions**
  A Hamartoma
  B Lymphoproliferative lesions
  C 'Tumorlet' (small-cell epithelial tumor)
  D Eosinophil granuloma
  E Sclerosing hemangioma
  F Inflammatory pseudotumor
  G Others

# MEMORIX SURGERY

## TNM classification of bronchial carcinoma

T1 Tumor that is 3.0 cm or less in greatest dimension, surrounded by lung or visceral pleura, and no bronchoscopically visible tumor in the main bronchus.

T2 >3 cm in greatest dimension
or: invasion of main bronchus ≤2 cm distal to the carina
or: tumor-associated atelectasis with obstructive inflammation up to the hilus
or: infiltration of the visceral pleura

T3 Invasion of the main bronchus <2 cm distal to the carina (carina not invaded)
or: infiltration of one of the following structures: chest wall, diaphragm, mediastinal pleura, parietal pericardium
or: tumor-associated atelectasis with obstructive disease of the whole lung

T4 Infiltration of one of the following structures: mediastinum, heart, great vessels, trachea, vertebral column, carina
or: malignant pleural effusion

N1 Ipsilateral peribronchial invasion and/or ipsilateral hilar nodes

N2 Ipsilateral mediastinal invasion and/or subcarinal lymph nodes

N3 Invasion of the contralateral lymph nodes
or: invasion of the scalene or supraclavicular lymph nodes

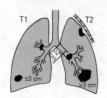
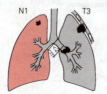
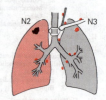

# HEART AND THORAX SURGERY

## Lung surgery procedures

**Classical resection**
Pneumonectomy
Lobectomy (right upper, middle or lower lobe)
(left upper or lower lobe)

Upper bilobectomy (right upper and middle lobes)
Lower bilobectomy (right middle and lower lobes)

**Bronchoplasty and vascular plastic resection** (conserving parenchyma)
**Atypical carcinoma and wedge resection**
**Exploratory thoracotomy** (thoracotomy to check operability)
**Diagnostic thoracotomy** (thoracotomy for doubtful findings)
**Open-lung biopsy** (in diagnosis of a diffuse lung disease)

**Standard intubation technique**

**Carlens' tube**
(for right-sided resection)

**White's tube**
(for left-sided resection)

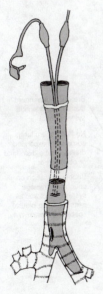
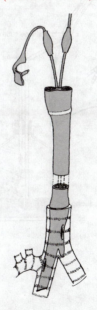

## MEMORIX SURGERY

### Thoracic drainage
**Indications**
Pneumothorax
Pyopneumothorax
Pyothorax (empyema)
Pleural effusion
Hemothorax
Chylothorax

(in **tension pneumothorax** the emergency treatment is needle puncture in the 2nd or 3rd intercostal space in the midclavicular line – converting the tension pneumothorax to an externally open pneumothorax.

**Chest tube insertion**
Standard approach: in the midaxillary line at nipple level

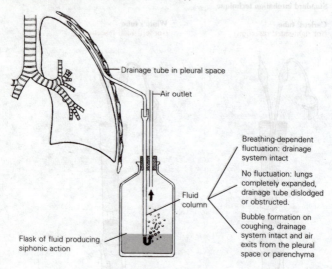

- Drainage tube in pleural space
- Air outlet
- Fluid column
- Flask of fluid producing siphonic action

Breathing-dependent fluctuation: drainage system intact

No fluctuation: lungs completely expanded, drainage tube dislodged or obstructed.

Bubble formation on coughing, drainage system intact and air exits from the pleural space or parenchyma

# HEART AND THORAX SURGERY

## Classification of mediastinal tumors
(Recommendations of the German Society for Surgery, 1980)

### 1 Autonomic mediastinal tumors

a. Tumors arising from mesenchymal connective tissue
   **Chondroma, fibroma, lipoma, myoma, myxoma, sarcoma, xanthoma, mixed types**
b. Tumors arising from the mediastinal blood and lymph vessels
   **Hemangioma, lymphangioma**
c. Primary mediastinal carcinoma

### 2 Fissural tumors and cysts

a. **Dermoid cysts, epidermoid cysts, teratoma cysts**
b. **Chorionepithelioma**

### 3 Cysts of dispersed origin

a. Mesothelial cysts
   **Pericardial cysts, pleural cysts**
b. Stem system
   **Enteric cysts**
   **Bronchogenic cysts**

### 4 Invasion from neighboring organs

a. Neurogenic tumors
   From interstitial tissue: **neurinomas, spindle cell sarcoma**
   From ganglion cells: **ganglioblastoma, ganglioneuroma, glioma, neuroblastoma**
   From sympathetic chain: **sympathioblastoma, sympathiogonioma**
   Paraganglioma: **pheochromocytoma, chemodectoma**
b. From the esophagus: **leiomyoma**
c. From the trachea: **cylindroma**
d. From the endocrine system: dystopic thyroid tumors, dystopic parathyroid gland tumors
e. Thymus tumors

### 5 Seminoma

a. Germ cell tumor
b. Carcinoid
c. Benign and malignant teratoma

### 6 Mediastinal tumors of generalized tumor formation

a. Malignant lymphoma
b. Hemoblastoma
c. Metastases of other malignancies

# MEMORIX SURGERY

## Mediastinal tumors: differential diagnosis

**Superior mediastinum**
Aortic arch
Superior vena cava
Brachiocephalic vein
Phrenic nerve
Vagus nerve
Left recurrent laryngeal nerve
Sympathetic trunk
Thoracic duct
Lymph nodes
Esophagus
Thymus
Trachea

**Anterior mediastinum**
Thymus
Lymph nodes
Connective fat tissue

**Posterior mediastinum**
Descending aorta
Intercostal arteries, veins, and nerves
Azygos vein/hemiazygos vein
Splanchnic nerves
Vagus nerves
Sympathetic trunk
Thoracic duct
Esophagus

**Middle mediastinum**
Pericardium and heart
Ascending aorta
Pulmonary artery
Superior and inferior vena cava
Pulmonary veins
Phrenic nerves
Pericardiophrenic artery
Pericardiophrenic vein

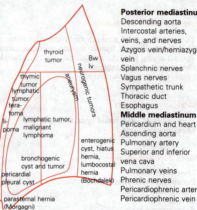

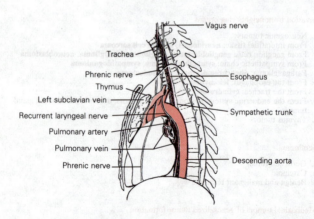

# HEART AND THORAX SURGERY

## Pleural effusion: differential diagnosis
(From Loddenkemper *et al.*, 1982)

Transudate (T) <30 g/l albumin (Alb)
Exudate (E) >30 g/l albumin
chyle (c), hemorrhagic (h), purulent (p), serous (s)

| Etiology/group | Disease | Look for | Alb |
|---|---|---|---|
| Oncostatic/hydrostatic | Cardiac insufficiency | s | T |
| | Constrictive pericarditis | s | T |
| | Liver cirrhosis with ascites | s | T |
| | Hypalbuminemia | s | T |
| | Salt retention syndrome | s | T |
| | Peritoneal dialysis | s | T |
| | Hydronephrosis | s | T |
| | Nephrotic syndrome | s | T |
| Infection | Tuberculosis | shpc | E |
| | Viral and mycoplasma | s(h) | E |
| | Parapneumonia | s(h) | E |
| | Unspecific empyema | p(s) | E |
| | Fungi and parasites | s(h) | E |
| Neoplastic diffuse malignancies | Mesothelioma | s(h) | E(T) |
| | Metastases from extrathoracic growths | shc | E(T) |
| | Bronchial carcinoma | shc | E.T |
| | Lymphoma and leukemia | shc | E.T |
| | Localized pleural tumors | shc | E.T |
| | Chest wall tumors | sh | E |
| | Accompanying melanomas | s | E.T |
| Vascular | Lung infarct | hs | E.T |
| | Cirrhosis | hs | E.T |
| Autoimmune | Rheumatoid arthritis | sc | E |
| | Systemic lupus erythematosis | s(h) | E |
| | Sjögren syndrome | s | E |
| | Mixed connective tissue disease | s | E |
| ABDC | Pancreatitis, pseudocyst | s(h) | E(T) |
| | Subphrenic abscess | sp | E |
| | Cirrhosis with ascites | s(h) | T(E) |
| | Abdominal tumor and ascites | s | T |
| | Meig's syndrome | s | T(E) |
| | Cholothorax (gallbladder fistula) | g | E |
| | Endometriosis | h | E |
| Traumatic | Hemothorax | h | E |
| | Chylothorax | c | T(E) |
| | Rupture of esophagus | P | E |
| | Operation (thorax, abdomen) | sh | ET |
| | Seropneumothorax | s(h) | E |
| Various | Uremic pleuritis | s(h) | E |
| | Myxedema | s | T |
| | Yellow nail syndrome | s(c) | E |
| | Postmyocardial infarct syndrome | s(h) | E |
| | Periarteritis nodosa | s | E |
| | Sarcoidosis | s(h) | T(E) |
| | Familial Mediterranean fever | s | E |
| | Benign asbestosis | s(h) | E |
| | Medication-induced | s | E |
| | X-ray pleural effusion | s(h) | E |
| | Lymphangiomatous | c | T(E) |
| | Tuberous sclerosis | c | T(E) |
| | Cholesterin-pleuritis (pseudo-chylothorax) | c | TE |
| | Intrapleural infusion | s(h) | ET |
| | Idiopathic | s(h) | ET |

### Diagnostic procedures
- Pleural aspiration
- Pleural punch biopsy
- Thoracoscopic and probe–excision for histologic examination

## Hemoptysis/hematemesis: diagnosis

| Hemoptysis | Hematemesis |
|---|---|
| Alkaline | Acid (offensive) |
| Mostly light red (frothy) | Mostly dark red–black (hematin, coffee-grounds, bright if massive or esophageal bleeding) |
| Admixed with sputum | Mixed with meal contents |
| Stools normal (except for swallowed blood) | Dark-stained stools (animal stool) |
| History: respiratory disease | History: gastrointestinal disease |

**Diagnostic procedures in blood-stained expectoration**
(Recommendations of the German Society for Pneumology and Tuberculosis, 1987)

| Occurrence of blood-stained expectoration |
|---|

1 Inflammatory diseases
 Tracheitis
 Acute bronchitis
 Exacerbated chronic bronchitis
 Bronchiectasis
 Tuberculosis
 Bacterial pneumonia
 Lung abscess
 Aspergillosis – mycetomatosis
 Echinococcal cysts

2 Neoplasia
a) Malignant growths
 Bronchial carcinoma
 Bronchus adenoma
  • Carcinoid
  • Adenocystic carcinoma
 Invasive mediastinal and esophageal tumors
 Malignant lymphoma with or without lung parenchyma affected
 Metastases
b) Benign tumors

3 Cardiovascular diseases
 Pulmonary embolus and infarct
 Left-heart failure
 Mitral stenosis
 Primary pulmonary hypertension
 Ruptured aortic aneurysm
 Rare heart defects
 Vascular anomalies
  • acquired (e.g. cirrhosis of liver)
  • congenital (e.g. A–V fistula)
 Veno-occlusive disease

4 Trauma
 Chest injuries
  • Lung contusion
  • Bronchial rupture

5 Foreign-body aspiration

6 Systemic diseases
 Vascular:
  • Wegener's granulomatosis
  • Goodpasture syndrome
  • Periarteritis nodosa
  • Idiopathic lung hemosiderosis
 Sarcoidosis
 Lung fibrosis, histiocytosis X
 Hemorrhagic diathesis

7 Iatrogenic bleeding
 Anticoagulant
 Streptokinase
 Urokinase
 Needling, biopsy

8 Anomalies
 Lung sequestration
 Lung endometriosis
 Broncholithiasis
 Cysts, bullae
 Cystic fibrosis, Osler's disease

9 Unclear

**Diagnostic measures**
- History, physical examination, exclude extrapulmonary bleeding (nose, pharynx, larynx, mouth, food passages, stomach). Site localization. Age (40 years: – bronchiectasis, open tuberculosis; 40 years – bronchial carcinoma, chronic bronchitis). Quantity of blood (considerable, light red – tuberculosis, aspergillosis; recurrence, little – tumor). Color (red-brown – pneumococcal pneumonia). Odor (foul) – lung abscess. Pain (lung infarct, trauma)
- Laboratory investigations: exclude blood coagulation disorders, delimit inflammatory, malignant and systemic processes
- Thoracic X-rays (tomography, CT, esophageal swallow), lung scintigraphy, pulmonoangiography, bronchial arterioangiography (embolization), bronchoscopy, bronchography

# HEART AND THORAX SURGERY

## Chest pain/differential diagnosis

**Pleural**
Pleuritis
Pleurodynia
Pleuropneumonia
Pleural tumor
Pneumothorax

**Pulmonary**
Pulmonary embolism
Pulmonary infarct
Pneumonia

**Mediastinal**
Mediastinitis
Mediastinal emphysema

**Gastrointestinal**
Hiatus hernia
Esophagitis
Boerhaave syndrome
Perforated esophagus
 (foreign body,
 iatrogenic)
Stomach–duodenal ulcer
Cholelithiasis
Cholecystitis
Cholangitis
Pancreatitis
Gastrointestinal tumor
Functional upper
 abdominal pain

**Psychogenic**
Fear
Neurotic
Hyperventilation

**Myocardial**
Angina pectoris
Cor pulmonale
Aortic stenosis or
 insufficiency
Mitral valve prolapse
Myocardial ischemia
Functional
Heart complaints

**Pericardial**
Pericarditis
Trauma

**Aortal**
Aneurysm dissecting

**Musculoskeletal**
Costochondrodynia
Thoracic wall tumor
Tietze's syndrome
Fractured rib
Contused rib
Sliding rib syndrome
Myositis
Herpes zoster
Precordial spasm
Intercostal neuralgia

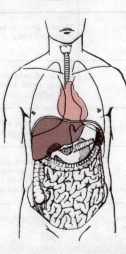

## Chest injuries

| Injury | Treatment |
|---|---|
| Pneumothorax<br>Hematothorax<br>Chylothorax | Thoracic drainage until complete re-expansion of the lung lobes |
| Open pneumothorax (mediastinal flutter) | Intubation, bandaging with three sides of bandage taped down, followed by chest tube placement |
| Tension pneumothorax | Needle puncture and conversion, followed by chest tube placement |
| Penetrating lung injury | Shock treatment, thorax drainage. Wound revision and thoracotomy if needed (e.g. hematothorax with blood loss over 300 ml/h over 3 h or 1500 ml initially) |
| Injuries of the great vessels, the heart, the pericardium<br>Heart tamponade<br>Trachea, bronchus injury<br>Massive, persistent bleeding<br>Massive endobronchial bleeding<br>Esophageal bleeding<br>Diaphragmatic injury<br>Open pneumothorax | Primary thoracotomy (Glinz, 1985) |

# HEART AND THORAX SURGERY

## Pulmonary embolus

**Definition**: embolic closure of one or more pulmonary artery branches

### Etiology
- Thrombosis (e.g. proximal limb vein thrombosis)
- Postoperative period, immobilization, confinement-to-be
- Immobilization in plaster for fracture or dislocation
- Association with ovulation inhibitors (birth control pills)
- Nicotine
- Absolute arrhythmia
- Myocardial infarct, insufficiency, valve defect
- Debilitating disease (chronic infection, malignancy)

### Differential diagnosis of chest pain

### Symptoms
- Sudden worsening of the general condition
- Sudden pain, sudden dyspnea, irritable cough
- Arrhythmia, tachycardia, tachypnea
- In infarct: chest pain, pleural rub, hemoptysis
- Anxiety, perspiration, consciousness disorder

### Clinical findings
- Arrhythmia, tachycardia, tachypnea, cyanosis
- Distended neck veins, enlargement of liver, jugular venous pulse
- Accentuated pulmonary sounds
- Heart sounds affected
- Rhonchi, rales, pleural rub, pleural effusion (if infarct)

### Laboratory findings
Fall in $PaO_2$, respiratory alkalosis

### ECG
- P pulmonale
- Arrhythmia, extrasystoles
- Right bundle branch block (complete or incomplete)
- ST lowering or raising
- T-inversion (negative in III, aVF, II)
- $S_1Q_{III}$-type

### Chest X-ray
- Often nonspecific
- Heart enlarged (right ventricle, right atrium, azygos vein, vena cava)
- Distention of the pulmonary arteries
- Sudden vascular rupture, peripheral clearing, wedge-shaped shadow
- Small amount of pleural effusion, atelectases, elevation of diaphragm

### Lung scintigraphy
- Perfusion deficit (confirm diagnosis with same-side ventilation scintigraphy)

### Pulmonary angiography
- Diagnostic confirmation (for indication of thrombolysis or thrombectomy; an indwelling catheter can be inserted for thrombolytic treatment)

## MEMORIX SURGERY

| Stage | Diagnosis | Aim of therapy | Treatment |
|---|---|---|---|
| 1 Normal pressure in circulatory systems | Chest X-ray ECG Blood-gas analysis Perfusion Scintigraphy Phlebography | Recurrence prophylaxis | Heparinization later replaced with oral anticoagulants, e.g. for 3 months after the event, for 12 months after one recurrence, for life after two recurrences For the duration of the risk with congenital anti-thrombin III deficiency or protein-C deficiency |
| 2 Hypotension, raised central venous and pulmonary artery mean pressure (25 mmHg) | Pulmonary angiography | Rapid relief of right ventricle | Thrombolytics (e.g. streptokinase, urokinase, rt-PA (recombinant tissue plasminogen activator), insertion of local or indwelling catheter or systemic i.v. |
| 3 Fulminating lung embolus, unstable circulation despite catecholamine treatment | Pulmonary angiography | Rapid restoration of circulatory stability, relieving the right ventricle | Embolectomy |

**Contraindications to anticoagulants**
- Gastrointestinal bleeding
- Intracerebral bleeding
- Bacterial endocarditis
- Proliferative retinopathy

**Indications for preventive operations in pelvic vein thrombosis (i.e. vena cava filters)**
- Recurrence under anticoagulant treatment
- Contraindications to anticoagulants
- Recurrent thromboembolism despite taking anticoagulants
- After embolectomy

# BREAST SURGERY

## Breast tumors, mastopathy and abscesses

### Congenital anomalies of the breast
- Absence of breast
- Supernumerary nipples or breasts
- Accessory axillary breast tissue (may be confused with tumor)
- Inversion of nipple

### Differential diagnosis of breast tumors
- Cyst
- Fibrosis
- Epithelial hyperplasia
- Sclerosing adenosis
- Fibroadenoma (most common)
- Phylloides tumor
- Intraductal papilloma
- Carcinoma
- Sarcoma (fibro-, lipo-, myxo-, chondro-, angio-, osteogenic sarcoma)
- Malignant lymphoma

### Baker classification of capsular contracture
(secondary to breast implant)
I   Augmented breast feels as soft as an unoperated breast
II   Breast feels less soft, implant can be palpated but is not visible
III   Breast feels firmer, implant can be palpated and is visible
IV   Breast feels cold and hard, is tender, distortion of implant is visible

### Infections
- Galactocele
- Acute mastitis (most common during lactating period)
- Mammary duct ectasia (plasma cell mastitis)
- Focal fat necrosis
- Abscess (see figure below, classification by localization)

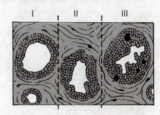

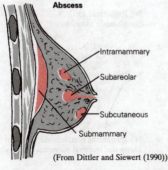

**Abscess**
- Intramammary
- Subareolar
- Subcutaneous
- Submammary

(From Dittler and Siewert (1990))

# MEMORIX SURGERY

## Breast cancer

### Diagnosis
Physical examination, mammography, sonography, tumor marker CA 15-3, fine-needle aspiration, needle biopsy, bone scan.

| Breast-conserving operation (lumpectomy) ||
|---|---|
| Indication | Contraindication |
| Tumor <2 cm | Multifocal carcinoma<br>Inflammatory carcinoma<br>Diffuse suspect microcalcification<br>Unfavorable tumor-to-breast proportion<br>Large adipose breast |

**Technique**: short approach to the tumor, curved concentric incision in dermal line, separate approach for axillary exploration between pectoralis major and latissimus dorsi muscles.

### Alternative treatment types
- Modified radical mastectomy (spares pectoral muscle)
- Homogeneous percutaneous postoperative radiation (after a breast-conserving operation)
- Adjuvant chemotherapy (in selected cases)
- Adjuvant hormone therapy (tamoxifen) in the post-menopause with positive hormone receptor finding
- Adjuvant treatment is mostly directed to prolongation of recurrence-free intervals

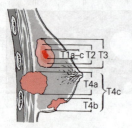

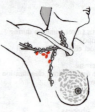

N1 Ipsilateral axillary lymph node invasion

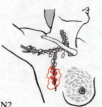

N2
Ipsilateral lymph node invasion with fixation of lymph nodes to one another or to other structures

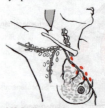

N3 Ipsilateral lymph node invasion along the internal mammary artery

## VISCERAL SURGERY

## Esophagus: differential diagnosis of dysphagia

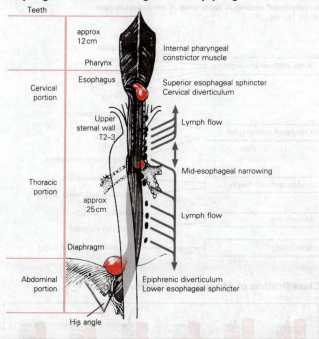

| Dysphagia | |
|---|---|
| **Oropharyngeal** | **Esophageal** |
| Goiter<br>Tumor (benign, malignant)<br>Anomaly<br>Diverticulum<br>Cerebrovascular disorder<br>Parkinson's disease<br>Multiple neuromuscular diseases<br>Scleroderma<br>Aganglionosis | Peptic stenosis<br>Esophageal tumor (benign, malignant)<br>Mediastinal tumor<br>Bronchial carcinoma<br>Adhesions<br>Stricture (caustic, reflux)<br>Compression (vascular anomaly, aortic aneurysm)<br>Schatzki's ring (distal esophageal stenosis at the transition site of squamous and columnar epithelium in hiatus hernia) |

## Esophagus: atresia

**Investigational methods in clarification of esophageal diseases**
(From Haring (1990))

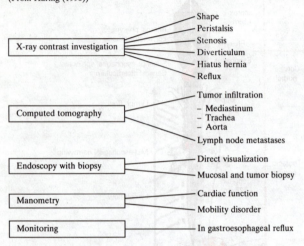

## Classification of esophageal atresias (Voigt)

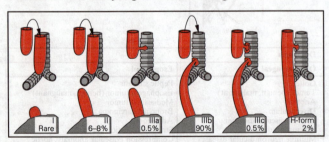

# VISCERAL SURGERY

## Esophagitis and diaphragmatic hernia

### Classification of esophagitis (after Savary and Miller, 1976)

I    Single or multiple superficial mucosal erosions with erythema and/or exudate
II    Confluent mucous membrane erosions
III    Mucous membrane erosions of the entire esophageal circumference (no spontaneous restitution)
IV    Chronic changes: ulcer with scar formation, stenosis, wall fibrosis, columnar cell scars, brachyesophagus

### Complications of esophagitis

- Peptic stenosis
- Endobrachyesophagus (distal esophagus covered with metaplastic (columnar) epithelium)
- Ulceration in the epithelial transition border (frequent)
- Barret ulcer in the endobrachyesophagus (rare)
- Secondary brachyesophagus after intrathoracic shrinkage (perifocal fibrosis)
- Malignant degeneration

### Different diaphragmatic hernias

|  |  | Operative indication |
|---|---|---|
| a) Developmental failure (His angle raised) | Asymptomatic → | None |
| b) Sliding hernia | Symptomatic → | For failed conservative treatment. For complications with bleeding, stenosis, endobrachyesophagus (Stenosis can often be dilated) |
| c) Paraesophageal hernia | | The possibility of complications such as bleeding, perforation incarceration |
| d) Upside-down stomach | | |
| Mixed type | | The possibility of complications through the paraesophageal portion |

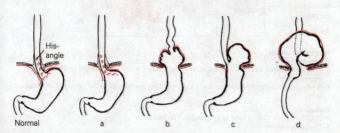

Normal     a     b     c     d

## Esophageal tumors
**Histologic classification of esophageal tumors (WHO, 1977)**

A Epithelial tumors
  I Benign
     1. Squamous epithelium papilloma
  II Malignant
     1. Squamous epithelium carcinoma
     2. Adenocarcinoma
     3. Adenocystic carcinoma
     4. Mucoepidermoid carcinoma
     5. Adenosquamous carcinoma
     6. Undifferentiated carcinoma
     7. Small-cell
        Oat cell carcinoma

B Non-epithelial tumors
  I Benign
     1. Leiomyoma
     2. Others
  II Malignant
     1. Leiomyosarcoma
     2. Others

C Different tumors
  I. Carcinosarcoma
  II. Malignant melanoma
  III. Others

D Secondary tumors

E Unclassified tumors

F Tumor-like changes
  I. Heterotopic
  II. Congenital cyst
  III. Fibrovascular polyp
       (fibrous polyp)

**TNM classification of esophageal carcinoma**

| | |
|---|---|
| T1 | Infiltration of the lamina propria or submucosa |
| T2 | Infiltration of the muscularis propria |
| T3 | Infiltration of the adventitia |
| T4 | Infiltration of adjacent structures |
| N1 | Invasion of regional lymph nodes |

**Surgical treatment**
**Curative:**
- Thoracoabdominocervical esophagectomy for tumors in the middle third (with left thoracotomy)
- Abdomino-transmediastinal-cervical esophagectomy for tumors in the proximal or distal third

**Palliative:**
- Endoscopically placed tube (e.g. Celestin, Haring)
- Bypass operation

## VISCERAL SURGERY

## Diaphragmatic foramina, common sites of defects

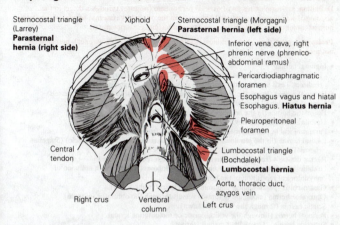

## Pelvic floor with localization of possible sites of hernia

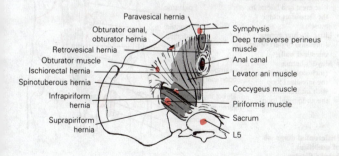

# MEMORIX SURGERY

## Hernia

**Definition:** sac-form extrusion of parietal peritoneum (rupture) through a defect in the abdominal wall coverings (external hernia) or in the mesentery (internal hernia) of facultative hernial contents (e.g. bladder, small and large intestine, great omentum)

**Prolapse:** descent through a peritoneal defect (e.g. postoperative dehiscence), herniation is not present

- Inguinal hernia
  (direct – exit medial to the epigastric vessels, mostly acquired)
  (indirect – exit lateral to the epigastric vessels, mostly congenital)
- Femoral hernia (below the inguinal ligament, mostly medial to the femoral vessels)
- Ventral (incisional) hernia
- Epigastric hernia (in the linea alba between xiphoid and umbilicus)
- Umbilical hernia (wide naval ring)
- Paraumbilical hernia (normal-size naval, separate from bulge)
- Lateral hernia (in the semilunar line lateral to the rectus abdominalis muscle) (Spigelian hernia)
- Rectus diastasis (relative operative indication, high recurrence rate)
- Umbilical cord hernia, omphalocele (fetal developmental defect with omission of physiological reposition of the bowel)
- Gastroschisis (paraumbilical abdominal wall defect, right > left)
- Obturator hernia (along the obturator vessels through the obturator foramen)
- Sciatic hernia (through the ischial foramen)
- Perineal hernia (through the vesicouterine or rectouterine space)
- Superior hernia – Grynfeltt–Lesshaft (through the upper triangle between the 12th rib and the erector spinae muscle)
- Inferior lumbar hernia – Petit's hernia (above the iliac crest and lateral to the latissimus dorsi muscle)
- Littré–Richter hernia (inclusion of part of the intestinal wall)
- Maydl's hernia (inclusion of more of the intestinal loop with incarceration of the abdominal loop)

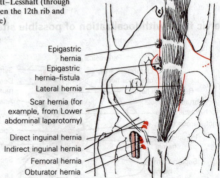

Epigastric hernia
Epigastric hernia–fistula
Lateral hernia
Scar hernia (for example, from Lower abdominal laparotomy)
Direct inguinal hernia
Indirect inguinal hernia
Femoral hernia
Obturator hernia

**Differential diagnosis of umbilical hernia–fistula:**
- Paraumbilical hernia
- Omphalocele, umbilical cord hernia
- Gastroschisis
- Patent omphaloenteric duct
- Urachus fistula

## VISCERAL SURGERY

## Diagrammatic anatomy of the inguinal region

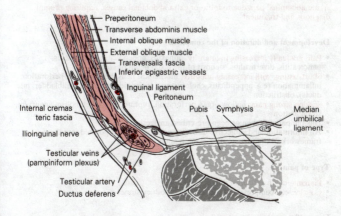

- Preperitoneum
- Transverse abdominis muscle
- Internal oblique muscle
- External oblique muscle
- Transversalis fascia
- Inferior epigastric vessels
- Inguinal ligament
- Peritoneum
- Pubis  Symphysis
- Median umbilical ligament
- Internal cremasteric fascia
- Ilioinguinal nerve
- Testicular veins (pampiniform plexus)
- Testicular artery
- Ductus deferens

**Caution:** testicular atrophy following an operation for inguinal hernia is the most common complication.

## Localization and relative incidence of internal hernias
(From Ghahremani and Meyers (1975))

- Foramen of Winslow (8%)
- Paraduodenal (53%)
- Transmesenteric (8%)
- Paracecal (13%)
- Supravesical (7%)
- intersigmoidal (6%)

# MEMORIX SURGERY

## Acute abdomen

### Definition

Acute abdominal pain due to intra- or extra-abdominal causes, requiring prompt diagnosis and treatment.

### Development and duration of the complaint

- Pain gradually increasing in intensity: adnexitis, appendicitis, cholecystitis, pancreatitis, diverticulitis, stenosis of the distal ileum or colon
- Short-lasting, with increasing intensity: mechanical ileus, hollow organ perforation, inflammation (e.g. appendicitis, cholecystitis), colic (kidney, ureter, gallbladder, bile ducts), obstruction
- Sudden strong pain: hollow organ perforation, rupture, arterial embolism/aneurysm, strangulation
- Has the patient taken or been prescribed analgesics?
- All information and subjective description should be incorporated into the framework of the general clinical impression of the case

### Type of pain

- Piercing: e.g. from perforation
- Colicky: e.g. compression by gallstones or kidney stones

### Unspecific symptoms

- Loss of appetite, retching, vomiting, fever, diarrhea, constipation, nausea, altered bowel habit, stool admixture, dehydration

### Preoperative

### Vascular or cardiac diseases

### Earlier similar complaints

### Physical examination

Body posture of patient (legs drawn up, doubled up, restless), flat respiration, blood pressure, pulse, signs of shock, temperature, lips/cheeks/mucous membranes (abnormal pigmentation; Addison's disease, Peutz–Jeghers syndrome), gums (lead deposition), skin (pigmentation, petechial hemorrhages, collagenosis), pupillary reaction (tabes dorsalis), ocular pressure (glaucoma), meningismus, cold perspiration, pallor, cyanosis, surgical scars, auscultation (heart, lungs [arrhythmia, pneumonia, pleural effusion, pneumothorax], peripheral pulses), bimanual palpation of abdomen ([liver, spleen], hernias, guarding, often an operative indication), verification of bladder filling, pressure and/or guarding, rigidity in the flank, rectal and genital examination, auscultation (peristaltic obstruction, 'deadly silence')

# VISCERAL SURGERY

**Ultrasound investigation**
Liver (parenchymal changes, size), gallbladder and bile ducts (stone, hydrops, thickening of wall), aorta (diameter, calcification, aneurysm), pancreas (enlargement, pseudocysts), kidneys (stones, capsular scarring, parenchymatous changes), urinary bladder (filling capacity), free fluid (e.g. in Morrison's pouch).

**X-ray general abdominal check**
Free gas under the diaphragm (Caution: ask about recent laparotomy/laparoscopy, tubal insufflation) → perforation of the gastrointestinal tract, subphrenic abscess, Chilaiditi's syndrome (interposition of colon between liver and spleen and diaphragm), rarely gas-producing peritonitis (repair in the left lateral position to better demonstrate the gas), repeat again after 1 hour
Free subhepatic air, pericecal, retroperitoneal
Free gas in the bile ducts (perforation)
Flatulence in stomach, ileum, colon (for ileus recognition)
Concrements, calcification
 Pancreas
 Gallbladder
 Kidney
 Urinary tract
 Vessels
 Echinococcal cyst
Size of kidney
Size of liver
Size of spleen
Psoas shadow

**Chest-X-ray, standing or sitting**
Air under the diaphragm, pleural effusion, pneumothorax, parenchymal infiltration, variations in cardiac configuration

**Laboratory tests**
Red and white blood cell count, determination of the clotting parameters, electrolytes, urine, creatinine, blood sugar, liver tests, amylase, blood gases

**ECG**

**Extra-abdominal causes of an acute abdomen**
**Cardiovascular**: myocardial infarct (particularly posterior wall infarct), acute right-heart insufficiency with liver congestion), periarteritis nodosa, pericarditis, lupus erythematosus
**Toxic**: food material, lead, arsenic, plant poison, medication (acetyl salicylic acid, butazolidine), fungi, mercury, thallium, alcohol
**Pulmonary**: pulmonary embolus, basal pneumonia, pneumothorax, pleurisy
**Metabolic**: diabetic precoma, hyperparathyroidism, acute intermittent porphyria, familial hyperlipidemia, Addison's disease, hypercalcemia, hyponatremia, Mediterranean fever
**Urologic**: acute retention of urine (e.g. in prostatic hypertrophy)
**Neurologic**: epilepsy, psychosis, herpes zoster, tabes dorsalis
**Hematologic**: leukemia, hemolytic anemia, polyglobulinemia, polycythemia
**Others**: acute glaucoma, Bornholm disease (Coxsackie), infectious mononucleosis, Schönlein–Henoch purpura
**Gynecologic**: ectopic pregnancy, pregnancy complication, fulminating adnexal tumor, postpartum pneumoperitoneum

# MEMORIX SURGERY

### Epigastrium
Pleurisy
Pericarditis
Myocardial infarct
Rectus sheath hematoma (e.g. postoperative)
Hiatus hernia, esophagitis
Boerhaave's syndrome, esophagus perforation (iatrogenic, foreign body)
Gastritis, gastric and duodenal ulcer
Pyloric stenosis
Cholelithiasis, cholecystitis, cholangitis
Pancreatitis
Upper small intestinal ileus, gastrointestinal tumor
Functional upper abdominal pain

### Right upper abdomen
Duodenal ulcer
Cholecystitis
Cholangitis
Cholelithiasis
Pancreatitis
Subhepatic, subphrenic abscess
Pyelonephritis

### Right lower abdomen
Appendicitis
Meckel's diverticulitis
Regional enteritis
Ileocecal tumor
Tuboadnexitis
Ovarian cyst
Ectopic pregnancy
Urolithiasis
Urinary tract infection
Incarcerated hernia

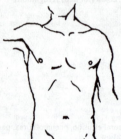

### Left upper abdomen
Pancreatitis
Splenic vein thrombosis – infarct
Subphrenic abscess
Pyelonephritis
Small bowel embolism

### Left lower abdomen
Diverticulitis
Tuboadnexitis
Ovarian cyst torsion
Ectopic pregnancy
Urolithiasis
Urinary tract infection
Endometriosis
Colitis
Incarcerated hernia

### Mid-abdomen
Appendicitis
Tuboadnexitis
Ovarian cyst (pedicle torsion)
Ectopic pregnancy
Rectus sheath hematoma (e.g. postoperative)
Adhesions
Ileum volvulus
Gastroenteritis
Metabolic disorders (diabetes mellitus, porphyria)
Urinary tract infection
Acute urinary retention
Incarcerated hernia
Small bowel embolism

## VISCERAL SURGERY

# Peritonitis

**Definition**
Localized or diffuse serofibrinous or purulent infection of the peritoneal cavity with organ manifestation involving the whole body via toxic damage to vital organ function (Wachsmuth, 1965; Haring, 1982)

**Symptoms**
Pain, guarding, protective posture (drawn up legs, bent back, dehydration, leukocytosis, tachycardia, shock, meteorism, vomiting, ileus (absent peristalsis, paralysis, fever, drowsiness, no passage of flatus)

**Causes**
A bacterial infection (e.g. pancreatitis), local toxic reaction with secondary bacterial invasion
Injury to bowel wall (e.g. ischemia, from mechanical ileus), infection of the peritoneum by direct invasion through the damaged bowel wall
Bowel perforation, with direct contamination
Bacterial infection (e.g. appendicitis, cholecystitis), infection crossing organ limits

**Sequelae**
Exudation, edema, minimal bleeding, hypovolemia, inflammation, increased vascularity, circulatory stress, toxemia, local intraperitoneal necrosis, paralytic ileus, endotoxic shock, fibrin deposition, adhesions

**Treatment**
(Feifel, G. and Gaitrasch, A. (1983))

### Immediate treatment of general peritonitis

| Procedures | Diagnostic | Treatment |
|---|---|---|
| Immediate<br>Central venous catheter<br>Stomach tube | Blood specimen for:<br>Red and white blood count<br>Electrolytes<br>Total albumin<br>Creatinine<br>Blood sugar<br>Platelets<br>Quick test<br>Amylase<br>Central venous pressure<br>Cross-match | Water–electrolytes–albumin and erythrocyte replacement<br>Antibiotics<br>Stress ulcer prophylaxis |
| ECG<br>X-rays:<br>  thorax<br>  abdomen<br>Arterial blood specimen | Blood gases | Digitalization if indicated<br><br>Intubation and artificial respiration if indicated |

### Supplementary measures if sepsis is suspected

|  | Diagnostic | Treatment |
|---|---|---|
| Citrated blood | Blood culture<br>Fibrinogen, fibrinomere<br>Bleeding time | Correction of specific disorders e.g.:<br>Factor replacement, heparin |
| Pulmonary artery catheter | Cardiac output/index<br>Peripheral vascular resistance<br>Pulmonary artery pressure | Inotropes<br>Vasopressors<br>Volume replacement<br>Cortisone |

**Operative treatment**
Early operation, basic cleansing, removal of fibrin deposits
Bacterial elimination, generous lavage

# MEMORIX SURGERY

## Ileus

### Definition
Disorder of intestinal motility
   mechanical (ileum, colon)
   functional (spastic, paralytic)
   mixed type

### Diagnosis
### History
Symptoms: (nausea, vomiting abdominal distention, constipation), depending on the localization of the disorder (e.g. vomiting early with normal stool habit, high ileus, distended abdomen with empty rectal ampulla, deep-seated ileus), preoperative consideration of the possibility of malignant disease (wasting, change in stool habit), medication (laxatives, antidepressants, medication for Parkinsonism), metabolic diseases (diabetes mellitus, uremia)

### Physical examination
Presence of a hernia, resistance, guarding, tension, inflation percussion note, 'deathly silence' as sign of paralytic ileus on auscultation, splashing sounds in mechanical ileus

**Rectal examination**: (filling of the rectal ampulla, tenderness in pouch of Douglas, size and consistency of the prostate)

### Abdominal X-ray examination
- Small bowel flow-through to demonstrate the intestinal loops
- Colon – contrast enema

### Preoperative procedures
Chemical-laboratory emergency diagnostic measures (e.g. erythrocytes, hemoglobin, hematocrit, leukocytes, Quick test, sodium, potassium, chloride, creatinine, liver screen, blood sugar, blood type), with extensions for special requirements
Blood gases (acid–base equilibrium) – particularly in severe cases
Central venous access – surveillance of central venous pressure, volume replacement
Stomach – ileal intubation, bladder catheter

### Treatment
#### Conservative
Stomach–intestinal intubation
Rectal enema
Control of cause

#### Operative treatment
Intervention after due consideration of the history, preoperative findings, age of the patient, etc.
Orientation with the anatomic and pathological circumstances
Mechanical decompression of the intestine
Removal of the cause of the ileus (e.g. adhesions, hernial orifice closure in incarcerated hernia, partial intestinal resection for wall ischemia with necrosis, tumor resection with attention to oncologic principles)
Adjustment of the intestinal loops and other abdominal contents

## VISCERAL SURGERY

## Ileus: frequency related to age and cause

| Cause | Perinatal | 1 | 5 | 10 | 20 | 30 | 40 | 50 | 60 | 70 | 80 | 90 |
|---|---|---|---|---|---|---|---|---|---|---|---|---|
| Intestinal atresia | × | | | | | | | | | | | |
| Intestinal stenosis | × | | | | | | | | | | | |
| Meconium ileus | × | | | | | | | | | | | |
| Congenital megacolon | × | × | | | | | | | | | | |
| Annular pancreas | × | × | | | | | | | | | | |
| Bowel duplication | × | × | | | | | | | | | | |
| Hypertrophic pyloric stenosis | × | × | | | | | | | | | | |
| Hirschsprung's disease | × | × | × | | | | | | | | | |
| Idiopathic intussusception | | × | × | | | | | | | | | |
| Meckel's diverticulum | | × | × | × | | | | | | | | |
| *Ascaris* infection | | | × | × | | | | | | | | |
| Foreign body | | | × | × | | | | | | | | |
| Adhesions | | | × | × | × | × | × | × | × | × | × | × |
| Incarcerated hernia | | × | × | × | × | × | × | × | × | × | × | × |
| Crohn's disease | | | | × | × | × | × | × | × | | | |
| Ulcerative colitis | | | | | | | × | × | × | | | |
| Volvulus | | | | | × | × | × | × | | | | |
| Carcinoma of colon | | | | | | | × | × | × | × | × | × |
| Stenosis from diverticulitis | | | | | | | | × | × | × | × | × |
| Mesenteric vascular thrombosis | | | | | | | | × | × | × | × | × |
| Gallstone ileus | | | | | | | | | × | × | × | × |
| Fecal impaction | | | | | | | × | × | × | × | × | |
| Age in years | Perinatal | 1 | 5 | 10 | 20 | 30 | 40 | 50 | 60 | 70 | 80 | 90 |

# MEMORIX SURGERY

## Elective ulcer surgery

**Indications for elective surgical treatment of gastric ulcer**
- Suspicion of malignancy
- Multiple ulceration
- Recurrent ulcer
- Giant ulcer
- Basic disease requiring the long-term administration of analgesics or antipyretics
- An anticipated rise in the mortality of a serious progressive second disease (e.g. chronic obstructive lung disease)

**Johnson's classification of gastric ulcer**

I    High-situated lesser curvature ulcer, hypo-acidity, an increasing reflux of bile acids and lysolecithin and disturbance of the microcirculation of the gastric mucosa

II    Gastroduodenal combination ulcer, hypersecretion through release of gastrin as a result of antral distension in pyloric stenosis (Dragstedt's mechanism)

III    Pre-/intrapyloric ulcer, hypersecretion; possible cause of gastric emptying disorder

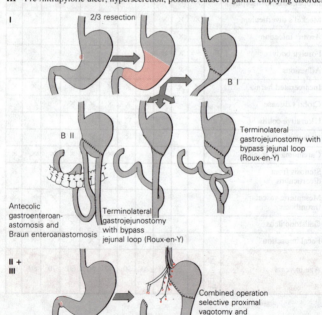

# VISCERAL SURGERY

## Duodenal ulcer

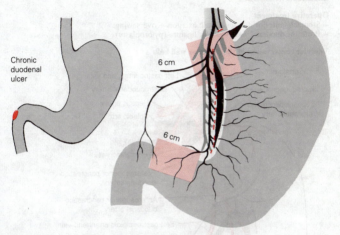

SPV (selective proximal vagotomy)

## Acute hemorrhage/perforated ulcer

**Treatment**
Endoscopic hemostasis

**Operative treatment**
- Stomach, anterior duodenal wall: excision + oversewing
- Posterior duodenal wall: vascular ligature (pyloroplasty)

**Vascular conservation of the posterior wall bulb**

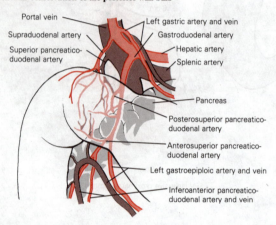

**Incision for unknown source of bleeding**
(After Esser, G. and Altmeier, G. (1990))

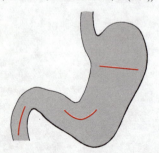

# VISCERAL SURGERY

## Classification of gastric carcinoma

**Pre-malignant carcinoma**
(limited to mucosa and submucosa)
Classification after the Japanese Society for Gastroenterological Endoscopy, 1962

**I** Arched type

**II** Superficial type

**IIa** Elevated

**IIb** Even

**IIc** Depressed

**I** Circumscribed solitary, polyposis
Carcinoma without raised ulceration

**II** Ulcerated carcinoma with sharp borders

**III** Ulcerated carcinoma, not well defined from adjacent tissue. Spreading by diffuse infiltration

**IV** Infiltrating carcinoma

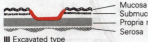

— Mucosa
— Submucosa
— Propria muscularis
— Serosa

**III** Excavated type

### Histologic classification (Lauren)

|  | Polypoid type | Infiltrating type |
|---|---|---|
| Horizontal tumor extension | Limited | Diffuse |
| Infiltration depth |  |  |
| Lymph node metastases | Rare | Frequent |
|  | Less extensive | Extensive |
| Curability | Frequent | Rare |
| Staging | Favorable | Unfavorable |

### TNM classification of gastric carcinoma

T1 Infiltration of the lamina propria or the submucosa
T2 Infiltration of the muscularis propria or the subserosa
T3 Infiltration of the visceral peritoneum (serosa)
T4 Infiltration of neighboring structures

N1 Invasion of lymph node ≤3 cm from the wall of the primary tumor
N2 Invasion of lymph nodes ≥3 cm from the edge of the primary tumor, with invasion of lymph nodes along the left gastric artery, common hepatic artery, splenic artery or the celiac trunk
(Invasion of the retropancreatic, para-aortal or paraesophageal lymph nodes or lymph node invasion of the hepatoduodenal ligament)

## Stomach: vessels and lymph nodes

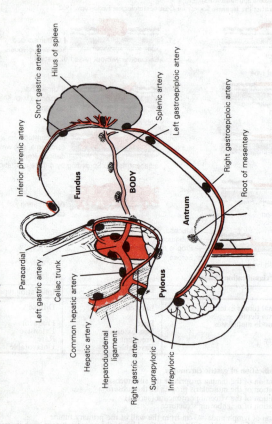

## VISCERAL SURGERY

# Surgery for gastric carcinoma: common procedures

### Resection
Subtotal: 4/5 of the stomach, greater omentum, lymphadenectomy (cardia spared)
Gastrectomy: stomach, greater omentum, lymphadenectomy
Extended gastrectomy: additional resection of neighboring organs, e.g. spleen, tail of pancreas, transverse colon, left lobe of liver

### Post-gastrectomy reconstruction
Jejunal interposition (Longmire–Gütgemann) (1)
Jejunal elevation with wide Braun anastomosis (Hoffmann) (2)
Terminolateral esophagojejunostomy with bypass Roux loop (3)
Artificial stomach formation with jejunal plication (Stewert and Peiper) (4)
Jejunal plication and reconstruction with Roux loop (Schreiber and Eichfuss) (5)

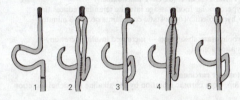

### To provide restitution of possible nutritional enteral function
Gastroenterostomy with Braun anastomosis (1), retrocolic (2)
Percutaneous endoscopic gastrostomy (PEG) (3)
Endoscopic tube implantation (Celestin, Haring), e.g. for inoperable cardia carcinoma (4)

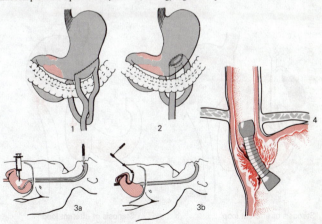

# MEMORIX SURGERY

## The operated stomach

**Recurrence after vagotomy/resection**
Incomplete vagotomy
Retained antral mucosa in remaining stomach
Retained antral mucosa in the duodenal stump
Pyloric stenosis
Gastrinoma
Hyperparathyroidism
Zollinger–Ellison syndrome

**Dumping syndrome (e.g. after B-II or Roux-en-Y anastomosis)**
Early dumping: rapid hyperosmolar food passage into the jejunum reduces the circulatory volume → hypovolemia (orthostatic complaints occur 30 minutes following a meal)
Late dumping: rapid carbohydrate absorption → increased insulin secretion → hypoglycemia 2 hours after a meal

**Stump carcinoma (anastomotic carcinoma)**
10–20 years after resection, from chronic irritation by the alkaline duodenal secretion

**Afferent loop syndrome**

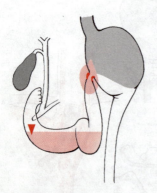

Stenosis of afferent loop

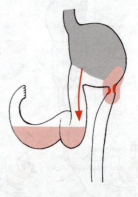

Stenosis of efferent loop

# VISCERAL SURGERY

# Small intestine: absorption and malabsorption

### Absorption areas of the small intestine

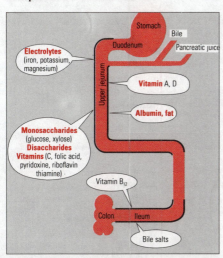

### Surgical significance of the malabsorption syndrome

Blind loop syndrome
Post-gastrectomy syndrome
Pancreatitis
Post-pancreatectomy
Small bowel inflammation (e.g. Crohn's disease)
Small bowel fistula (e.g. enterocutaneous, enterocolic)
Mesenteric tumor
After extended small bowel resection
After proctocolectomy with installation of an ileostoma

### Diagnosis of the malabsorption syndrome

Weight of stool, fat content
Absorption tests: ($B_{12}$ serum concentration, Schilling's test, D-xylose loading test), glucose tolerance test, lactulose test, iron loading
Function tests (gastric secretions analysis, pancreatic ferments, radioiodine test)
Endoscopy and biopsy (ileum biopsy, rectal biopsy)
Hormone levels determined, immunoelectrophoresis, 5-hydroxyindole-acetic acid
X-ray examination (abdomen, e.g. pancreatic calcification)

## MEMORIX SURGERY

# Small intestine procedures
## Resection of diverticulum

Lifting the diverticulum

Transverse closure

### Partial enterectomy

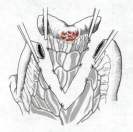

Specimen showing course of the vascular arcades

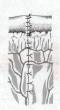

Demonstration of an end-to-end anastomosis. Closure of mesenteric slit (preserving the vessels)

### Common ileal anastomoses

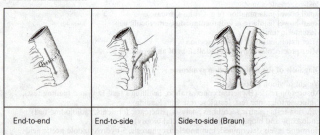

| End-to-end | End-to-side | Side-to-side (Braun) |

## VISCERAL SURGERY

## TNM classification of colorectal carcinoma

T1 Infiltration of the submucosa
T2 Infiltration of the muscularis propria
T3 Infiltration of the subserosa, i.e. the non-peritonealized pericolic or perirectal tissues
T4 Perforation of the visceral peritoneum, i.e. infiltration of other organs or structures

N1 Metastases in 1–3 pericolic or perirectal lymph nodes
N2 Metastases ≥4 pericolic or perirectal lymph nodes
N3 Metastases in lymph nodes along a named vascular trunk

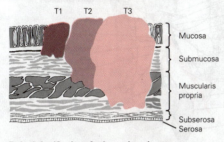

## Dukes' classification of colorectal carcinoma

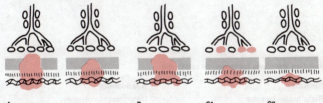

**A**
Tumor limited
to bowel wall

**B**
Tumor penetrating
bowel wall,
lymph nodes free

**C1**       **C2**
Invasion of lymph nodes
○ tumor-free lymph nodes
● lymph nodes with metastases

## Localization and relative frequency of colorectal carcinoma

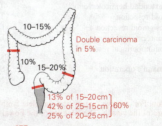

10–15%

10%

15–20%

Double carcinoma
in 5%

13% of 15–20 cm ⎫
42% of 25–15 cm ⎬ 60%
25% of 20–25 cm ⎭

### Diagnosis
– Colonoscopy
– Rectoscopy
– Digital examination

# MEMORIX SURGERY

## Standard colorectal procedures

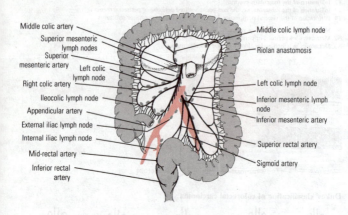

**Standard resections for colorectal carcinoma**

| Resection | Anastomoses |
|---|---|
| Right hemicolectomy | Ileotransversocolostomy |
| Right extended hemicolectomy | Ileotransversocolostomy |
| Transverse and flexure resection | Colocolostomy |
| Palliative partial transverse resection | |
| Left hemicolectomy | Transverse-transversocolostomy |
| Left extended hemicolectomy | Transverse-sigmoidostomy |
| Sigmoid resection | Transverse-sigmoidostomy |
| Rectosigmoid resection | Descending-rectal anastomosis |
| Low anterior resection | Descending-rectal anastomosis |
| Abdominoperineal resection | Sigmoid colostomy |
| | No anastomosis, perineal closure |
| Hartmann's operation | Sigmoid colostomy |
| | No anastomosis |

**Caution:** For curative surgery, the complete lymphatic bed should be excised after ligature of the vessels. The integrity of the bowel should be preserved throughout.

# VISCERAL SURGERY

## Artificial anus

|  | Ileostomy | Sigmoid colostomy |
|---|---|---|
| **Indication** | After proctocolectomy, e.g. for ulcerative colitis, granulomatous colitis, disseminated pre-malignancy (polyposis, Gardner's syndrome) | Deep-seated rectal carcinoma, anal carcinoma, stool incontinence, widespread fistula system in the region of the rectum or anal canal |
| **Localization** | Right lateral rectus sheath between navel and iliac ant. sup. spine: dependent on individual necessity (abdominal girth, skin folds) | Left lateral rectal wall between navel and ant. sup. iliac spine; dependent on individual necessity (abdominal girth, skin folds) |
|  | Caution: costal border, inguinal curve, skin folds, adiposity, ribs. demonstrated to patient<br>Later: possible cachexia from malignancy (reduction in abdominal girth) | |
| **Technique** | Stoma 6 cm above the skin level stretched and cuffed, fixation to peritoneum, plication of the last ileal loop.<br><br>**Accurate mucosal skin closure** | After the usual median laparotomy all the layers of the abdominal wall are grasped, pulled towards the midline and opened transversely.<br>**Caution: do not tear or stenose the extracted bowel, preserve vascular supply (danger of necrosis)**, fixation of bowel to skin only after cuffing |
| **Complications** | Skin erosion, dermatitis<br>Ileostomal fistula<br><br>Retraction, necrosis, prolapse, stenosis, parastomal hernia | |

## Complications

### Necrosis resulting from insufficient blood supply
Torsion of the recipient loop
Excessive preparation and ligature of the supplying vessels
Tension on the sutures through inadequate mobilization
Prolapse (an intra-abdominal supply loop that is too long)
Peristomal hernia (redundant supply loop, inadequate fixation to the lateral abdominal wall)

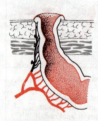
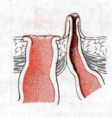

### Skin irritation

Irritating intestinal contents
Malfitting appliance

### Perforation

Iatrogenic from the irrigation catheter
Perforated diverticulum
Ulcer

### Stenosis/closure

Inadequate skin and/or fascial opening
Skin contraction
Indigestible food contents
Recurrent carcinoma

### Retraction

Insufficient mobilization

### Peristomal hernia

Raised intra-abdominal pressure
Excessive fascial opening
Redundant supply loop

### Fistula

Reaction to suture material
Crohn's disease

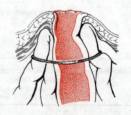

# VISCERAL SURGERY

## Gallstones

Around 20% of the inhabitants of Western industrial countries have gallstones.
Cholelithiasis causes the most complications – e.g. 'dyspepsia', pains, inflammation, stone migration, malignant degeneration.

**Risk factors**
- Obesity, cholesterol-rich nutrition
- Hormonal contraceptives
- Diabetes mellitus, hyperparathyroidism
- Ileocecal resection, Crohn's disease
- Chronic inflammatory disease

**Diagnosis**
- History, risk factors
- Sonography
- X-ray examination of abdomen
- Oral cholecystogram
- (Computed tomography, for localization and operability)
- Endoscopic retrograde cholangiopancreatography (ERCP) for combined diagnosis and treatment
- Percutaneous transhepatic cholangiography in special cases

**Specific preoperative diagnostic procedures**
- Gastroscopy (stomach, intestine)
- Colon investigation (tumor marker, colonoscopy, contrast X-ray enema)

**Complications**
- In cholecystolithiasis:
    Cholecystitis (acute, chronic), hydrops of gallbladder, empyema, gangrene, penetration, bilio-digestive fistula, gallstone ileus, gallbladder perforation, bile peritonitis, sepsis, liver abscess, subphrenic abscess, carcinoma of gallbladder
- In choledocholithiasis:
    Stenosis of ampulla, ampullary stricture, ampullary carcinoma, obstructive jaundice, purulent cholangitis
    Pancreatitis, biliary liver cirrhosis, bile duct carcinoma

**Treatment**
- 'Classical' cholecystectomy (and main bile duct examination)
- Endoscopic cholecystectomy
- Extracorporeal shock wave lithotripsy
- Transduodenal ampullary section with endoscopic operative stone extraction
- Medical dissolution of stones

**Operative indications in bile duct diseases**
- Malignancy, suspicion of malignancy
- Empyema of gallbladder or gangrene, acute cholecystitis
- Gallstone ileus
- Bile duct disease with peritonitis
- Acute biliary pancreatitis
- Obstructive jaundice
- Stenosis of the exiting bile ducts
- Symptomatic or long-standing cholecystolithiasis
- Porcelain gallbladder
- Septic gallbladder
- *Salmonella* elimination
- Mirizzi's syndrome

# MEMORIX SURGERY

## Carcinoma of the biliary system

### TNM classification of gallbladder carcinoma

- T1a Infiltration of the mucous membrane
- T1b Infiltration of the musculature
- T2 Infiltration of the perimuscular connective tissue
- T3 Infiltration of the serosa or of a neighboring organ (liver ≤2 cm)
- T4 Infiltration of the liver >2 cm or in ≥2 neighboring organs (stomach, duodenum, pancreas, omentum, extrahepatic, bile ducts)
- N1a Invasion of regional lymph nodes (of cystic duct, bile duct, hilus)
- N1b Invasion of regional lymph nodes (of head of pancreas, periduodenal periportal, celiac, superior mesentery)

### TNM classification of carcinoma of the extrahepatic bile ducts

- T1a Infiltration of the mucous membrane
- T1b Infiltration of the musculature
- T2 Infiltration of the perimuscular connective tissue
- T3 Infiltration of neighboring structures (liver, pancreas, duodenum, gallbladder, colon, stomach)
- N1a Invasion of regional lymph nodes (of cystic duct, bile duct, hilus)
- N1b Invasion of regional lymph nodes (of head of pancreas, periduodenal, periportal, celiac, superior mesentery)

### TNM classification of carcinoma of the ampulla of Vater

- T1 Limited to the ampulla of Vater
- T2 Infiltration of the duodenal wall
- T3 Infiltration of the pancreas ≤2 cm
- T4 Infiltration of the pancreas >2 cm
- N1 Invasion of regional lymph nodes

### Biliary–gastrointestinal anastomoses/bile drainage

Choledochojejunostomy
Hepaticojejunostomy (see figure)
Choledochoduodenostomy (side-to-side)
Cholecystojejunostomy
Hepatojejunostomy
Endoscopic bile duct catheter insertion (e.g. Tytgatt catheter)
Percutaneous transhepatic bile drainage
T-drain insertion

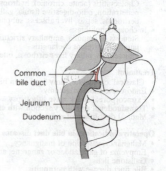

# VISCERAL SURGERY

## Liver: anatomy
**Functional anatomy of the liver (Coulinaud) with segments labeled**
(From Bismuth (1988))

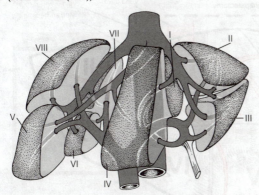

**Anatomic variations of the arterial blood supply of the liver**
(From Tung and Haring (1990))

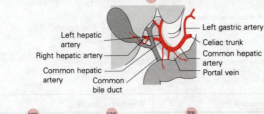

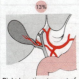

Right hepatic artery out of the superior mesenteric artery

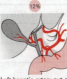

Left hepatic artery out of left gastric artery

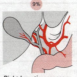

Right hepatic accessory artery out of mesenteric artery

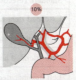

Left accessory hepatic artery from left gastric artery

# MEMORIX SURGERY

## Liver: standard resections

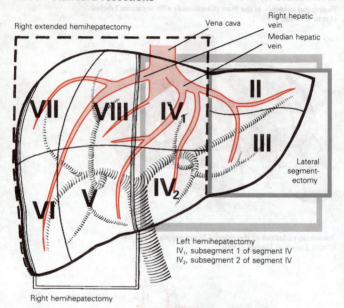

Right extended hemihepatectomy
Vena cava
Right hepatic vein
Median hepatic vein
Lateral segmentectomy
Left hemihepatectomy
IV$_1$, subsegment 1 of segment IV
IV$_2$, subsegment 2 of segment IV
Right hemihepatectomy

| Standard resection | Resected segments | |
|---|---|---|
| Extended right hemihepatectomy | V, VI, VII, VIII | I, IV |
| Right hemihepatectomy | V, VI, VII, VIII | |
| Left extended hemihepatectomy | II, III, IV | I, V |
| Left hemihepatectomy | | I |
| Lateral segmentectomy | II, III | |

## VISCERAL SURGERY

# Histologic classification of liver tumors

1. Primary tumors of epithelial origin
   Benign: Hepatocellular adenoma
   Bile duct adenoma
   Biliary cystadenoma
   Malignant: Hepatocellular carcinoma (most common related to hepatitis B and C)
   Biliary cholangiocarcinoma
   Combined hepatocellular and cholangiocarcinoma
   Hepatoblastoma
   Carcinosarcoma
   Undifferentiated carcinoma and unclassifiable tumors

2. Non-epithelial tumors
   Benign cavernous hemangioma
   Infantile hemangioendothelioma
   Hemangiosarcoma
   Embryonal carcinoma
   Lymphangioma

3. Metastatic tumors (especially colon, breast, lung and malignant melanoma)

4. Hematopoietic malignancies (that may invade the liver)
   Hodgkin's disease
   Non-Hodgkin's lymphoma
   Leukemia (acute and chronic)

5. Epithelial abnormalities and tumor-like lesions
   Liver cell dysplasia
   Bile duct abnormalities
   Hamartoma
   Congenital biliary cysts
   Focal nodular hyperplasia
   Nodular regenerative hyperplasia
   Hepatic peliosis
   Heterotopy
   Teratoma

### TNM classification of the primary hepatocellular and the intrahepatic bile duct carcinomas

T1 ≤2 cm, no vascular invasion
T2 ≤2 cm with vascular invasion
or multiple tumors ≤2 cm, no vascular invasion
T3 >2 cm with vascular invasion
or multiple tumors ≤2 cm, limited to one lobe, with vascular invasion
or multiple tumors, one of which limited to one lobe, with or without vascular invasion
T4 Multiple tumors in one lobe or tumor(s) with invasion of a large branch of the portal vein or the hepatic veins
N1 Regional lymph node metastases

# MEMORIX SURGERY

## Jaundice
### Classification
- Prehepatic – hemolytic anemia
- Hepatic – disordered bilirubin excretion from primary hepatocyte damage, 'medical' jaundice
- Posthepatic – obstruction of the extrahepatic bile ducts, 'surgical' jaundice

### Diagnostic procedures
- History
- Physical examination
- Laboratory investigations
- Sonography
- Abdominal X-rays
- Oral cholecystogram
- Hepatobiliary scan
- Endoscopic retrograde cholangiopancreaticography (ERCP) for suspicious posthepatic causes
- Percutaneous transhepatic cholangiography
- Computed tomography
- Angiography (mesenteric–celiac arteriogram)

| Differentiation | Intrahepatic | Posthepatic jaundice |
|---|---|---|
| Indirect bilirubin (serum) | + | ./. |
| Direct bilirubin (serum) | +, ++ | +, ++ |
| Alkaline phosphatase (serum) | + | ++, +++ |
| SGGT | +, ++ | ++, +++ |
| Urine color | Dark | Dark |
| Urine urobilinogen | Positive | Negative |
| Stool color | Pale | Pale |
| Serum GOT | +++ | +, ++ |
| Serum GPT | +++ | +, ++ |

### Jaundice – differential diagnosis
#### Intrahepatic
- Toxic hepatitis (alcohol, fungus)
- Infectious hepatitis (acute, chronic)
- Medication-induced hepatitis (contraceptives, halothane, tuberculostatics, cytostatics)
- Liver congestion
- Congenital liver fibrosis
- Liver cirrhosis (alcohol)
- Biliary atresia
- Sclerosing cholangitis
- Primary biliary cirrhosis
- Benign cholestasis
- Pregnancy jaundice
- Caroli's syndrome
- Liver tumor
- Metastasis
- Bile duct carcinoma
- Gallstones
- Lymphoma

#### Posthepatic
- Bile duct stone
- Mirizi's syndrome
- Bile duct stenosis, -stricture (inflammatory, congenital, postoperative)
- Tubal stenosis (in chronic pancreatitis)
- Ampullary stenosis
- Sclerosing cholangitis
- Parasitic bile duct obstruction
- Bile duct tumor (carcinoma, papilloma, cyst)
- Tumor of head of pancreas
- Ampullary tumor
- Metastases
- Lymphoma

## VISCERAL SURGERY

## Portal hypertension
**Causes:**

**High-volume pressure**      e.g. arterioportal fistula (iatrogenic, traumatic)

**High-resistance pressure**

Prehepatic:      e.g. thrombosis of portal or splenic vein
Tumor compression from adjacent organs

Intrahepatic:      Presinusoidal: e.g. biliary cirrhosis
Postsinusoidal: e.g. liver cirrhosis (95%)

Posthepatic (rare)      e.g. Budd–Chiari syndrome, venous occlusive disease

## Collateral circulation

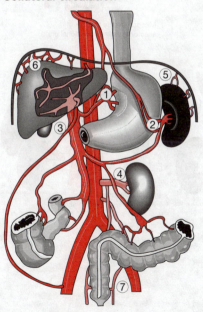

① Gastroesophageal anastomosis over the left gastric vein
② Anastomoses over the short gastric veins
③ Vascular junction between the left branch over the umbilical vein, paraumbilical veins and epigastric veins
④ Anastomoses between spleen and left renal vein
⑤ Collateral vessels between spleen capsule and diaphragmatic veins
⑥ Collateral joining between intrahepatic portal branches and diaphragmatic veins
⑦ Retroperitoneal collateral vessels to the paravertebral plexus of the vena cava

(From Haring and Hirner (1987))

## MEMORIX SURGERY

## Portal system shunt operations

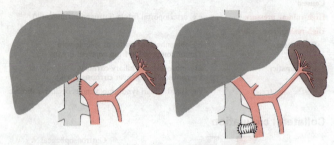

Portocaval end-to-end anastomosis

Mesocaval side-to-side anastomosis (interpositional graft)

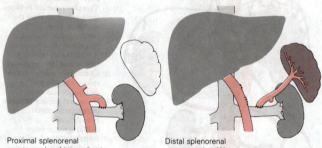

Proximal splenorenal anastomosis – Linton shunt

Distal splenorenal anastomosis – Warren shunt

## VISCERAL SURGERY

# Pancreas and pancreatitis

## Etiology
Alcohol-related and biliary causes (together >90%)
Common bile duct obstruction (stone, tumor, ampullary spasm), hyperlipidemia, hyperparathyroidism, infectious diseases, ulcerative colitis, tuberculosis, idiopathic, medication (e.g. azathioprim, furosemide, L-asparaginase, mercaptopurine, methyldopa, pentamine, procainamide, sulfonamide, tetracycline, thiazide diuretics, bleeding disorders, toxic, uremia)

**Revised Marseille classification of pancreatitis**
(From Sarles, Gry and Singer (1985))

### Acute pancreatitis
Clinical: acute one-sided abdominal pain, elevated pancreatic enzymes (blood, urine), generally favorable progress, occasional severe cases with shock, renal insufficiency, single attack or recurrent
Morphologically: mild (peripancreatic fat tissue necrosis, interstitial edema), severe (necrosis of fatty parenchymatous tissue, hemorrhages)
The clinical symptoms and the morphological condition do not always correspond. Disorders of pancreatic function vary in length and severity. Rarely is there a transition to a chronic form.

### Chronic pancreatitis
Clinical: recurrent persistent abdominal pain, with possible steatorrhea, diabetes
Morphologically: irregular sclerosis and permanent loss of endocrinal gland tissue. Dilatation of the pancreatic (Wirsung's) duct (stricture, stones, protein loss), focal necrosis, segmental/diffuse necrosis, calcification. Mostly irreversible loss of pancreatic function.

### Special forms
Obstructive chronic pancreatitis (tumor, scar), morphological and functional recovery are possible

### Complications
Progressive inflammation, abscess formation and necrosis, formation of pseudocysts, abdominal and intestinal bleeding

## Anatomy

# Pancreatic tumors

## Symptoms
Upper abdominal pain, weight loss

## Diagnosis
↑ Serum amylase, ↑ α-chymotrypsin in stools, ↑ CA 19-9, ↑ CA 50, sonography, angiography, ERCP, with biopsy (fine-needle aspiration)

## Histologic classification of pancreatic tumors (WHO, 1978)
I   Epithelial tumors
   A Benign
      1. Adenoma (papillary adenoma)
      2. Cystadenoma

   B Malignant
      1. Adenocarcinoma
      2. Squamous cell carcinoma
      3. Cystadenocarcinoma
      4. Acinous cell carcinoma
      5. Undifferentiated carcinoma

II   Islet cell tumors
III  Non-epithelial tumors
IV   Mixed tumors
V    Unclassified tumors
VI   Neoplasms of the hematopoietic and lymphatic systems
VII  Metastatic tumors
VIII Epithelial abnormalities
IX   Tumor-like changes

## TNM classification of exocrine pancreatic carcinomas
(duct adenocarcinoma, acinar cell carcinoma, cystadenocarcinoma)
T1a ≤2 cm
T1b >2 cm
T2  Infiltration of duodenum, bile ducts or peripancreatic tissues
T3  Infiltration of stomach, spleen, colon or adjacent large vessels
N1  Invasion of regional lymph nodes (see figure)

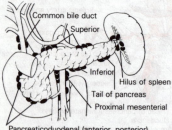

Common bile duct
Superior
Inferior
Hilus of spleen
Tail of pancreas
Proximal mesenterial
Pancreaticoduodenal (anterior, posterior)

# VISCERAL SURGERY

## Pancreas: standard operations

### Resections
- Distal resection (left resection) – resection of the pancreas tail and body to the crossing of the superior mesenteric vein (I)
- Subtotal pancreatectomy – resection with a small duodenal rest, duodenum and common bile duct remain preserved (II)
- Whipple's operation – resection of head of pancreas, duodenum, 2/3 of stomach, gallbladder and distal bile ducts; reconstruction by hepatojejunostomy, pancreaticojejunostomy, antecolic Braun anastomosis (III)

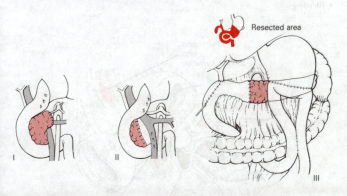

**Drainage operations** (e.g. for pancreatic pseudocysts or chronic pancreatitis)
- Cystojejunostomy with Roux–Y anastomosis (I)
- Laterolateral pancreaticojejunostomy Roux–Y anastomosis (after Puestom (II)
- Pancreatic tail resection with end-to-end pancreaticojejunostomy with Roux–Y anastomosis (after Du Val) (III)

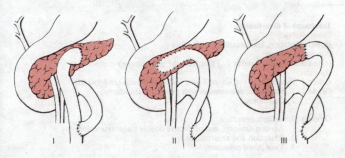

## Diverticulosis/diverticulitis of the colon
False diverticulum – mucosal prolapse through the musculature
Most common location – sigmoid colon

**Complications**
- Inflammation: covered perforation into the mesocolon or paracolon, peri-diverticular abscess, free perforation, peritonitis
- Fistula: enteroenteric, enterocutaneous, enterovesical, enterogenital
- Stenosis: ileus
- Bleeding

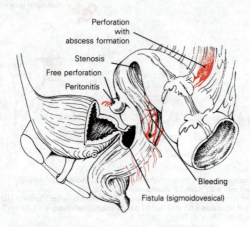

**Treatment of diverticulitis**
Conservative
Bowel regulation, laxatives/fiber, antibiotics
For complications
(extended abscess, stenosis ...) first treat the inflammatory component
Operative
Grade 1  Resection of the affected area and anastomosis (end-to-end)
Grade 2  1. Resection, anastomosis with protective colostomy
         2. Colostomy
         or
Grade 3  Schloffer's operation
         1. Abscess drainage and protective double transverse colostomy
         2. Resection and anastomosis
         3. Take down colostomy

## VISCERAL SURGERY

## Crohn's disease and ulcerative colitis

**Operative indications for Crohn's disease**

- High-grade stenosis, stricture
- Fistula (enteroenteral, vaginal, cutaneous, vesical ...)
- Abscess
- Ileus
- Massive bleeding
- Severe anal involvement with resultant incontinence
- Perforation, peritonitis
- Failure of conservative treatment

**Operative indications for ulcerative colitis**

- Proof of precancerous transformation
- Long-lasting course of the disease (increased risk of cancer)
- Toxic megacolon
- Massive hemorrhage
- Severe stenosis
- Perforation, peritonitis

| Crohn's disease | Ulcerative colitis |
|---|---|
| **No curative surgery possible**<br>• Conservative resection<br><br>• layered single end-to-end anastomosis<br><br>• no bypass anastomosis (except for duodenal invasion) | **'Curable' by proctocolectomy**<br>Liberal resection for carcinoma prophylaxis radical operation (proctocolectomy)<br><br>• only by radical operation (proctocolectomy) is it possible to preserve continence |

# MEMORIX SURGERY

## Spleen

**Examination methods**
- Bimanual palpation in right lateral position (size, consistency)
- Sonography (size, parenchymal changes, abscess, cyst, hematoma)
- Abdominal examination (limits, size, contour, calcification, displacement by neighboring structures such as stomach or left flexure)
- CT (abscess, trauma, cysts, tumors)
- Angiography (vascular abnormalities, trauma)

**Indications for splenectomy**
- Trauma (birth, traumatic rupture)
- Organic (abscess, tumor, cyst, vascular anomaly, splenic vein thrombosis, primary hypertrophy)
- Diseases of the blood or blood-forming system (malignant lymphoma, spherocytosis, thalassemia, elliptocytosis, sickle cell anemia, immunothrombocytopenic purpura, leukemic reticuloendotheliosis, chronic myeloid leukemia, myelofibrosis)
- Others (portal hypertension, for consideration in operations for malignant tumors)

**Results of splenectomy**
- Identify pathological cell types (acanthocytes, microspherocytes, target cells)
- Identify other cell types (Heinz bodies, Howell–Jolly bodies, basophil granulations)
- Elevated blood viscosity (raised risk of thrombosis)
- Transient thrombocytosis (indicates anticoagulant therapy)
- Persistent leukocytes
- Elevated immunoglobulin A and G
- Lowered immunoglobulin M
- Elevated postoperative infection rate (in 50% by *Strep. pneumoniae*, indicating administration of antibiotic 3–4 weeks preoperatively)
- Post-splenectomy sepsis

**Spleen preservation measures** (after partial resection)
- Parenchymal suture
- Laser coagulation
- Fibrin adhesion
- Inclusion in absorbent material

## VISCERAL SURGERY

## Abdominal arteries

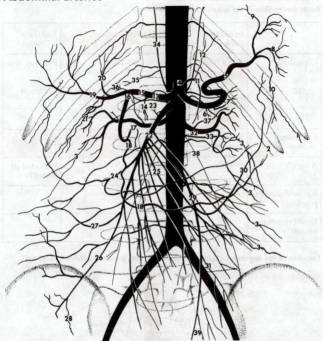

1. Intercostal artery
2. Subcostal artery
3. Lumbar artery
4. Celiac trunk
5. Splenic artery
6. Dorsal pancreatic artery
7. Great pancreatic artery
8. Splenic end branches
9. Short gastric
10. Left gastroepiploic artery
11. Left gastric artery
12. Esophageal branches from 11
13. Common hepatic artery
14. Right gastric artery
15. Proper hepatic artery
16. Gastroduodenal artery
17. Superior pancreaticoduodenal artery
18. Right gastroepiploic artery
19. Right ramus of proper hepatic artery
20. Left branch of proper hepatic artery
21. Cystic artery
22. Superior mesenteric artery
23. Inferior pancreaticoduodenal artery
24. Middle colic artery
25. Jejunal arteries
26. Ileocecal artery
27. Right colic artery
28. Branch for appendix
29. Inferior mesenteric artery
30. Left colic artery
31. Sigmoid artery
32. Renal artery
33. Renal accessory artery
34. Inferior phrenic artery
35. Superior suprarenal artery
36. Middle suprarenal artery
37. Inferior suprarenal artery
38. Testicular artery (internal spermatic or ovarian artery)
39. Superior rectal artery

(From Muller *et al.*)

## MEMORIX SURGERY

## Visceral arterial block
### Acute obstruction of the superior mesenteric artery

|  | Initial stage 1–6 h | Quiet interval 7–12(48) h | End stage >12(48) h |
|---|---|---|---|
| Clinical signs | Initial triad: 1. Abdominal pain 2. Signs of shock 3. Diarrhea (anoxia) | Tolerable, continuous Few local signs<br><br>Worsening of general condition<br><br>Bowel peristalsis disappears | Paralytic ileus<br><br>Peritonitis |
| Laboratory findings | Results negative | Increasing leukocytosis | |
| X-rays | Negative | Mostly negative | Increased air content |
| Revascularization possible | +++ | ++ | (+) |
| Bowel resection necessary | Average | + | ++ |

**Location of the important obstructive processes with possible collateral pathways**

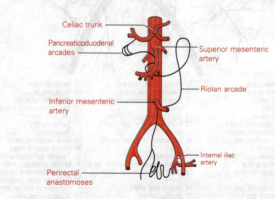

(From Volmar, J. (1982))

## VISCERAL SURGERY

## The retroperitoneum

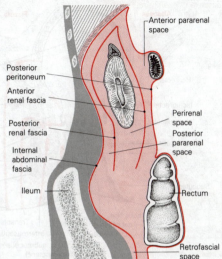

### Symptoms
- Palpable tumor
- Dull abdominal pain
- Weight loss, anemia
- Neurological effects

### Diagnosis
- Clinical examination (skin pigmentation from old hematoma, pressure or pain in the renal area, varicocele from renal carcinoma or obstructed venous return, edema of legs due to caval compression). Sonography (direct demonstration of an aortic aneurysm, a space-occupying fluid collection). Needle aspiration to confirm the diagnosis
- Abdominal examination (space occupation, displacement, psoas border)
- CT (direct confirmation, good prediction of extent), puncture for confirmation of diagnosis
- Angiography (differentiation of the course of the vessels in simple and malignant tumors – I.V. urography)
- Gastrointestinal contrast radiography – barium enema
- Lymphography

### Differential diagnosis
- Abscess
- Hematoma
- Retroperitoneal fibrosis [primary: Ormond's, secondary: after radiation, inflammatory, medication-induced (methysergine)]
- Trauma (duodenum, kidney, pancreas ...)
- Tumor (benign, malignant, metastatic)
- Spinal cord disease (injury)

## MEMORIX SURGERY

## Proctology: anal abscesses and fistulae

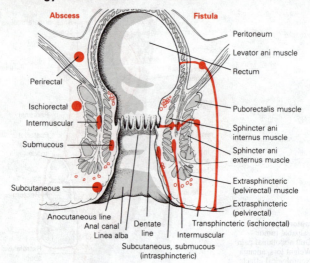

1. **Abscesses:** classification by localization

2. **Fistulae:** classification by localization
   Relation to sphincter
   Extent (complete, incomplete)

**Treatment**
For **1:** opening and drainage of abscess
For **2:** identification of fistula, splitting, excision (mostly at two sittings)

**Caution:** incontinence results after division of the internal sphincter and levator ani muscle

### TNM classification of anal carcinoma

T1 ≤2 cm
T2 ≤5 cm
T3 >5 cm
T4 Infiltration of neighboring organs (bladder, urethra, vagina)
N1 Invasion of perirectal lymph nodes
N2 Invasion of inguinal or internal iliac nodes of one side
N3 Invasion of perirectal and inguinal lymph nodes or bilateral internal iliac lymph nodes, or bilateral inguinal lymph nodes

# VISCERAL SURGERY

## Hemorrhoids

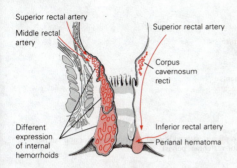

### Miles classification of internal hemorrhoids
I  Only visible proctoscopically
II  Prolapse – spontaneous reposition
III  Prolapse – manual reposition necessary
IV  Fixed prolapse – reposition not possible

### Anorectal diseases
1. Abscess/fistula: resulting from radiation, Crohn's disease, leukocytosis, lymphoma, pilonidal sinus, pyodermia fistulans, infection (spec. venereal), AIDS, malignancy, deformity, injury, idiopathic
2. Fissure: severe pain during and after defecation, digital examination painful and generally impossible. Usually at 6 o'clock
3. Hemorrhoids: usually at 3, 7 and 11 o'clock
4. Coccydynia: coccygeal pain of unclear origin
5. Cryptitis/papillitis: inflammation of Morgagni's crypts and anal papillae
6a. Proctitis
6b. Ulcerative coloproctitis
7. Stenosis/stricture
8. Tumors
    Anal papilla (hypertrophic)
    Bowen's disease
    Buschke–Löwenstein tumor
    Condylomata acuminata
    Dermoid cyst
    Eczema
    Venereal granuloma
    Carcinoma (squamous cell, adeno-)
    Malignoma (melanoma, neurogenic, sarcoma)
    Paget's disease
    Perianal thrombosis
    Prolapse (anus, rectum)
9. Injury (e.g. foreign body, accident)

# MEMORIX SURGERY

## Fractures

**Diagnosis**

1. Clinical examination
   a) Definite signs of fracture
      - Abnormal mobility
      - Deformity
      - Crepitus
      - Visible bone fragments
   b) Suggestive signs of fracture
      - Hematoma
      - Pain
      - Swelling
      - Tenderness

2. X-ray examination in two planes, with additional anterior/posterior and lateral/oblique views, CT (e.g. for vertebrae, pelvis)

**Treatment**

- Reduction
- Conservative, operative (stabilization)
- Rehabilitation

**Therapeutic procedures**

|  | Conservative | Operative |
| --- | --- | --- |
| Advantages | Operative and anesthetic risks avoided<br><br>No surgical scars | Rapid restoration of function to the injured extremity (AO principle)<br>• Anatomic reduction and stable bone repair → primary bone healing without callus<br>• Early activity, and joint mobilization<br><br>Reliable stabilization with conservation of vascularity → secondary bone healing (principle of biological bone fixation) |
| Disadvantages | Prolonged immobilization<br>Muscle atrophy<br>Possible joint stiffness<br>Increased risk of thrombosis and embolism | • Operative risks (damage to neighboring structures – blood vessels, nerves, ligaments), motion and/or sensory deficits, infection, scar formation<br>• Incompatibility, factors against physical applicability<br>• May require a second operation for removal of internal fixation |

## ORTHOPEDIC SURGERY

# Fracture healing
## Primary healing

**Assumption**
Anatomic repositioning of the fracture fragments
Elimination of motion at the fracture site

| Contact healing | Layered healing |
|---|---|
| Formation of a resorption channel (osteoclast)<br>Activation of the osteoblasts<br>Filling in with lamellar bone | Building up of the bone texture in lamellae |

**Secondary healing**

e.g. from movement at the fracture face
Resorption of the fracture surface
Callus formation in the fracture hematoma (fibroblastic)
Changes in the bone texture
Dysfunctional rebuilding process

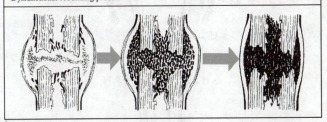

**Delayed healing**
Ischemia, avascular fracture fragments, infection, disturbance at the fracture line, sympathetic reflex dystrophy, insufficient callus formation, compartment syndrome, pseudoarthrosis (false joint formation)

**Pseudoarthrosis**
Hypertrophic: excess callus formation with no associated diminution in fracture stability
Oligotrophic: little callus formation, unstable fracture
Atrophic: no callus formation, no stability
Defect: lack of bone fragments

## MEMORIX SURGERY

# Duration of healing of different bone fractures

Average healing time in adults in **weeks**.
(After Schlosser (1968))

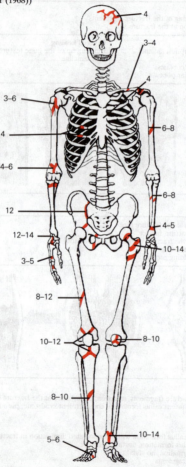

## ORTHOPEDIC SURGERY

# Immobilization in childhood

**Rules for average immobilization period for the most frequent injuries in childhood (in weeks)**
(From van Laer (1986))

|  | To 5 years | 5–10 years | >10 years |
|---|---|---|---|
| Clavicle | 1 | 2 | 2–3 |
| Humerus |  |  |  |
| – proximal stable | 1 | 1–3 | 2–3 |
| – proximal unstable | 1 | 2–3 | 3 |
| – mid-shaft | 2 | 3–4 | 4–6 |
| – supracondylar | 1–2 | 2–3 | 3–4 |
| – radial condyle | 3 | 3–4 | 4 |
| – ulnar condyle, Y-fracture | 2–3 | 3 | 3–4 |
| – ulnar epicondyle (+ elbow dislocation) | 2–3 | 2–3 | 3 |
| Proximal end of radius | 1 | 2 | 2–3 |
| Olecranon | 1 | 2–3 | 3–4 |
| Head of radius and elbow dislocation | – | 3 | 3 |
| Forearm shaft | 3 | 4 | 4–6 |
| Distal radius | 2 | 3–4 | 4–5 |
| Distal radial epiphysis dislocation | – | 2–3 | 3–4 |
| Wrist dislocation | – | 4–6 | 6–12 |
| Mid-hand subcapital and basal | – | 2 | 2–3 |
| – Shaft |  | 3–4 | 4–8 |
| Finger subcapital and base | 1–2 |  | 2–3 |
| – Shaft | 2–3 | 3–4 | 4–8 |
| Femur |  |  |  |
| – femoral head | – | 4–6 | 6–12 |
| – subtrochanteric | 3–5 | 4–5 | 4–6 |
| – shaft | 1–3 | 4–5 | 4–6 |
| – condylar | 2–3 | 3–4 | 4 |
| Tibia and leg |  |  |  |
| – eminences | – | 3–4 | 4–6 |
| – proximal metaphysis | 2–3 | 3–4 | 4 |
| – shaft | 2–3 | 3–5 | 4–6 |
| – supramalleolar and joint (ankle) | 2–3 | 3–4 | 4–5 |
| Heel and calcaneus | – | 4–8 | 6–12 |
| Mid-foot base and subcapital | 2–3 | 3 | 3–4 |
| Toes | 1 | 1–2 | 2–4 |
| Tibulotalar |  |  |  |
| – displaced bones | – | 3 | 3–4 |

Metaphyseal fractures heal about twice as quickly as diaphyseal fractures.
Transverse diaphyseal fractures heal more slowly than oblique ones.

## MEMORIX SURGERY

## AO classification of fractures: diagnostic coding
(From Muller, Allgower, Schneider and Willenegger (1992))

**Diagnostic coding**

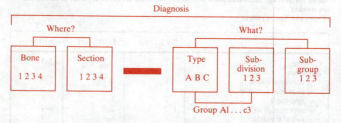

e.g. 32–B2.1 subtrochanteric wedge fracture of femoral diaphysis with inflexion wedge

| 3 | 2 | – | B | 2 | 1 |
|---|---|---|---|---|---|
| Femur | Diaphysis | | Wedge fracture | Inflexion wedge | Subtrochanter |

Localization (where?)    **Bone**
(1 . . .) humerus
(2 . . .) radius/ulna
(3 . . .) femur
(4 . . .) tibia/fibula

**Bone section**
(. . . .1) proximal
(. . . .2) diaphysis
(. . . .3) distal
(. . . .4) malleoli

Morphology (what?)    **Type** A, B, C

**Subdivision** 1, 2, 3

**Subgroup** 1, 2, 3

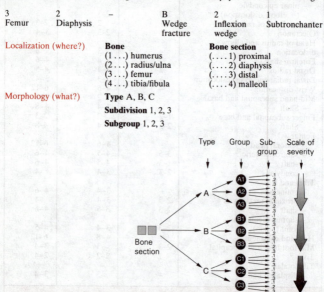

Please find further explanation and description of this classification in Muller *et al.* (1992).

# AO classification of fractures: humerus

## 11-Humerus proximal

### 11-A Humerus proximal ... extra-articular fracture

A1 ... tubercular
A2 ... metaphysis impacted
A3 ... metaphysis non-impacted

### 11-B Humerus proximal ... extra-articular bifocal fracture

B1 ... with metaphyseal impaction
B2 ... no metaphyseal impaction
B3 ... combined with scapulohumeral dislocation

### 11-C Humerus proximal, joint fracture

C1 ... little dislocated
C2 ... dislodged and impacted
C3 ... dislodged (dislocated)

## 12-Humerus diaphysis

### 12-A Humerus diaphysis, single fracture

A1 ... spiral
A2 ... oblique
A3 ... transverse

### 12-B Humerus diaphysis, wedge fracture

B1 ... wedge twist
B2 ... bent wedge
B3 ... fragmented wedge

### 12-C Humerus diaphysis, complex fracture

C1 ... spiral
C2 ... storied
C3 ... irregular

## 13-Humerus distal

### 13-A Humerus distal, extra-articular fracture

A1 ... apophyseal
A2 ... metaphysis simple
A3 ... metaphysis fragmented

### 13-B Humerus distal, partial joint fracture

B1 ... lateral-sagittal
B2 ... medial-sagittal
B3 ... frontal plane

### 13-C Humerus distal complete fracture

C1 ... simple articular simple metaphyseal
C2 ... simple articular, metaphyseal fragmented
C3 ... fragmented

# AO classification of fractures: radius/ulna

## 21-Radius/ulna proximal
21-A Radius/ulna proximal, extra-articular fracture

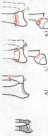

A1 ... ulna, radius intact
A2 ... radius, ulna intact
A3 ... both bones

21-B Radius/ulna proximal ... joint fracture of one bone

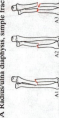

B1 ... articular fracture of ulna, radius intact
B2 ... of radius, ulna intact
B3 ... extra-articular of both

21-C Radius/ulna proximal. Joint fracture both bones

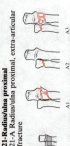

C1 ... simple
C2 ... one bone simple, the other fragmented
C3 ... fragmented

## 22-Radius/ulna diaphysis
22-A Radius/ulna diaphysis, simple fracture

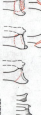

A1 ... ulna, radius shaft intact
A2 ... radius, ulna shaft intact
A3 ... both bones

22-B ... Radius/ulna diaphysis, wedge fracture

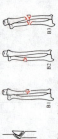

B1 ... of ulna, radius shaft intact
B2 ... of radius, ulna shaft intact
B3 ... of one bone, combined with one fracture of the other

22-C Radius/ulna diaphysis complex fracture

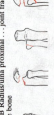

C1 ... of ulna, simple of radius
C2 ... of radius, simple of ulna
C3 ... both bones

## 23-Radius/ulna distal
23-A Radius/ulna distal, extra-articular fracture

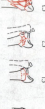

A1 ... ulna, radius intact
A2 ... simple and impacted
A3 ... radius, fragmented

23-B ... Radius/ulna distal: part joint fracture of radius

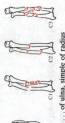

B1 ... sagittal plane
B2 ... dorsal slope (Barton)
B3 ... palmar slope (reversed Barton, Goyrand-Smith 11)

23-C Radius/ulna distal, complete joint fracture radius

C1 ... simple articular and metaphyseal
C2 ... simple articular, metaphyseal
C3 ... fragmented

# AO classification of fractures: femur

## 31-Femur proximal
### 31-A Femur proximal. Trochanter region fractures

A1 ... single pertrochanteric
A2 ... fragmented pertrochanteric
A3 ... intertrochanteric

### 31-B Femur proximal, femoral neck fracture

B1 ... subcapital, little displacement
B2 ... transcervical
B3 ... subcapital, displaced

### 31-C Femur proximal, fracture of head

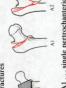

C1 ... pure split
C2 ... pure compression
C3 ... combination of two fractures

## 32-Femur diaphysis
### 32-A Femur diaphysis, simple fracture

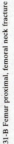

A1 ... spiral
A2 ... oblique
A3 ... transverse

### 32-B Femur diaphysis, wedge fracture

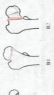

B1 ... twisted wedge
B2 ... bent wedge
B3 ... fragmented wedge

### 32-C Femur diaphysis, complex fracture

C1 ... spiral
C2 ... staged
C3 ... irregular

## 33-Femur distal
### 33-A Femur distal, extra-articular fracture

A1 ... single
A2 ... with metaphyseal wedge
A3 ... complex metaphyseal

### 33-B Femur distal, partial joint fracture

B1 ... unicondylar lateral sagittal
B2 ... unicondylar medial, sagittal
B3 ... frontal plane

### 33-C Femur distal, complete joint fracture

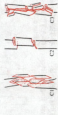

C1 ... simple articular metaphysis
C2 ... single articular, fragmented metaphysis
C3 ... fragmented

# AO classification of fractures: tibia/fibula

## 41-Tibia/Fibula, Tibia proximal
### 41-A Tibia proximal, extra-articular fracture

A1 ... abrasion
A2 ... single metaphyseal
A3 ... metaphyseal fragmented

### 41-B Tibia proximal, partial joint fibula fracture

B1 ... clean splitting
B2 ... clean compression
B3 ... compression with splitting

C1 ... single articular and metaphyseal
C2 ... single articular and metaphyseal fragments
C3 ... multi-fragmented

## 42-Tibia/Fibula, Tibia diaphysis
### 42-A Tibia diaphysis single fracture

A1 ... spiral
A2 ... oblique
A3 ... transverse

### 42-B Tibia diaphysis, wedge fracture

B1 ... twist wedge
B2 ... bent wedge
B3 ... fragmented wedge

C1 ... spiral
C2 ... staged
C3 ... irregular

## 43-Tibia/Fibula, Tibia distal
### 43-A Tibia distal, extra-articular fracture

A1 ... single metaphyseal
A2 ... with metaphyseal wedge
A3 ... complex metaphyseal

### 43-B Tibia distal, partial joint fracture

B1 ... clean split
B2 ... compression with fragmentation
B3 ... compression with fragmentation

C1 ... single articular and metaphyseal
C2 ... single articular and metaphyseal fragmented
C3 ... multi-fragmented

## 44-Tibia/Fibula, Malleoli
### 44-A Malleoli, lateral infrasyndesmal lesion

A1 ... isolated
A2 ... with medial malleolar fracture
A3 ... with posteromedial fracture

### 44-B Malleolar, transyndesmal fibula fracture

B1 ... isolated
B2 ... with added medial
B3 ... with added medial and Volkmann

C1 ... diaphyseal fibula-fragment fracture
C2 ... diaphyseal fibula fracture, fragmented
C3 ... proximal fibula

## ORTHOPEDIC SURGERY

## Epiphyseal fractures and growth

**Salter–Harris classification of epiphyseal fractures**

I   Epiphysiolysis
II  Epiphysiolysis with metaphysis wedge fracture
III Epiphysiolysis with epiphysis wedge fracture
IV  Epi- and metaphyseal fracture

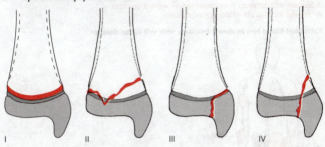

**Relative growth potential of individual epiphyses (%)**
(From van Laer (1986))

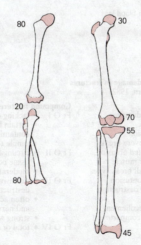

## MEMORIX SURGERY

## Open fractures and soft tissue damage
**Management of open fractures and fractures with significant soft tissue damage**
Constant observation and documentation of the peripheral circulation
Reduction at the site of accident
First dressing at the site of accident
First dressing change in the operating theater
Adequate débridement is essential before wound closure
A 'second look' is advisable before closure

**Estimated blood loss in closed fractures with soft tissue damage**

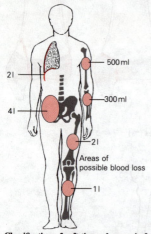

- 2 l
- 500 ml
- 300 ml
- 4 l
- 2 l
- Areas of possible blood loss
- 1 l

**Classification of soft tissue damage in fractures**
(after Tescherne and Oestern, 1982)

**Closed fractures**
Fr G 0
- little soft tissue damage single break

Fr G I
- superficial abrasion
- simple to mid-severe break

Fr G II
- deep contaminated abrasion, localized skin or muscle contusion with all break types

Fr G III
- extensive skin contusion skin crushing or destruction of muscle
- subcutaneous decollement
- decompensated compartment syndrome
- all fracture types

**Compound fractures**
Fr O I
- lacking or slight contusion
- certain bacterial contamination
- simple to mid-severe break

Fr O II
- circumscribed skin and soft tissue contusion
- moderate contamination

Fr O III
- extensive soft tissue destruction
- often accompanying vascular and nerve injury
- strong wound contamination

Fr O IV
- total or subtotal amputation

# ORTHOPEDIC SURGERY

## Conservative treatment of fractures

### Application of plaster bandaging
- Sparingly padded (but: bulky padding over joint projections, note course of vessels and nerves, e.g. peroneal nerve)
- Circular bandaging following contours and skin fissures
- Final survey on the circulation, mobility and sensation

### Typical traction sites
(in combination with plaster or splinting)

Skull calliper

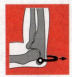
Olecranon

Supracondylar tibial tuberosity

Calcaneus

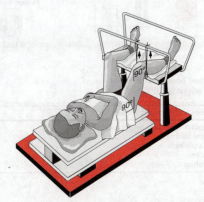
Weber table

Regular monitoring of motor function (traction, weighting, infection in the area of the traction pin) is an essential requirement

# Bone fixation methods

**Principles of the AO technique**
(From Muller, M.E. *et al.* (1977))

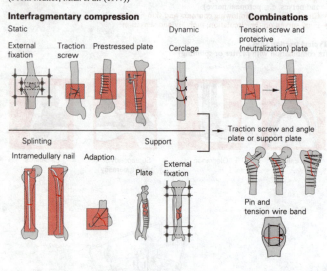

**Principles of 'biological' bone fixation**
(From Claudi and Oedekoven (1991))

| Reliable stabilization with vascular conservation |
|---|
| e.g.: – Limited contact–dynamic compression plate<br>– Solid marrow nailing<br>– 'Monorail' shift nails<br>– Clamp fixation<br>– Forceps fixation |

# ORTHOPEDIC SURGERY

## Fracture of radius

**Aim – reposition of the radius structure**
Restoration of the original radius length
Achievement of a correct axial position
Restoration of the joint surfaces

**Indications for the operative treatment of fracture of the radius**
Fragmented fracture/debris zone
Radio-ulnar separation
Ulnar dislocation
Danger of displacement (Smith's fracture – palmar fragment dislocation)

**Usual bone fixation procedures**
Wire fixation
Screw fixation
Plate fixation
External fixation

## Sympathetic reflex dystrophy (Sudeck dystrophy)
**Symptom triad:**

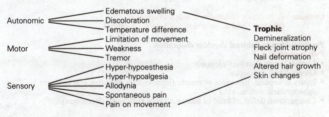

Autonomic
- Edematous swelling
- Discoloration
- Temperature difference

Motor
- Limitation of movement
- Weakness
- Tremor

Sensory
- Hyper-hypoesthesia
- Hyper-hypoalgesia
- Allodynia
- Spontaneous pain
- Pain on movement

**Trophic**
- Demineralization
- Fleck joint atrophy
- Nail deformation
- Altered hair growth
- Skin changes

### The symptoms are not uniform

Etiology   Trauma (independent of the degree of severity), plaster bandage, operation, nerve injury
Symptoms   Appearance of symptoms within hours to days after the initiating event
           Development of symptoms from minutes to hours
Progress   Acute stage (generally with a rise in temperature)
           Dystrophy stage (generally subnormal temperature)
           Stage of atrophy (irreversible changes)

### Treatment
Begin as soon as possible, otherwise a poor outcome is to be expected
Physiotherapy – below the pain threshold
Sympathetic block, plexus block
Systematic anti-inflammatory medication (cortisone, calcitonin, Ca-, β-blockers)
Psychological procedures (relaxation, bio-feedback, postural training)

# MEMORIX SURGERY

## Elbow or shoulder dislocation

### Hueter's triangle
- Equilateral triangle of 90° in flexion of the elbow joint (dorsal aspect)
- Disruption of the triangle is an indication of a fracture or dislocation

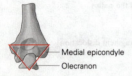
- Medial epicondyle
- Olecranon

### Dislocation of the head of the radius
- Mostly an injury of small children (Chassaignac)
- Reduction by rapid supination of the forearm

### Dislocation of the shoulder
Clinically: Empty joint socket, upper arm lightly abducted ('feathered')
X-rays: In two planes

Caution: A posterior dislocation is easily overlooked
(the arm fixed in adduction and internal rotation)

### Predisposition to habitual shoulder dislocation
**Post-traumatic:**
- Limbus injury (Bankart's lesion)
- Glenoid wall deficiency
- Injury to capsule, ligaments or muscle (intermediate glenohumeral ligament, subscapularis muscle, etc.)
- Compression defect of head of humerus (as in Hill–Sachs depression)

**Constitutional:**
- Glenoid dysplasia
- Unfavorable inclination of glenoid
- Dysplasia of head of humerus
- Diminished retroversion of the proximal humerus

# ORTHOPEDIC SURGERY

## Shoulder

**Differential diagnosis of shoulder–arm pain**
(After Mumenthaler (1980))

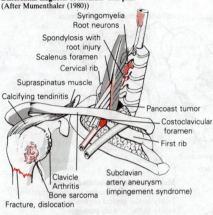
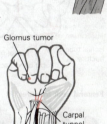

**Tossy classification of acromioclavicular joint injury**
I: Stretching of the acromioclavicular ligaments
II: Tearing of the acromioclavicular ligaments
III: In addition tearing of the coracoclavicular ligaments

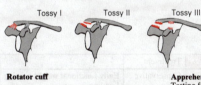

### Rotator cuff

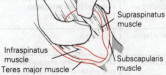

### Apprehension test
Testing for instability by abduction of 90% and forced external rotation; positive in anterior dislocation through pressure of the left thumb

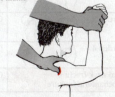

# Fractures of the pelvis, hip joint and femoral neck
## Pelvic and hip joint fractures

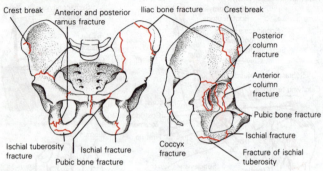

**Most commonly associated injuries**
Retroperitoneal vascular injuries/hematoma
Injury to the genital organs
Injury to the urinary passages
Rectal injury
Nerve injuries
Injuries to the peritoneum and its contents

### Femoral neck fractures

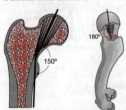

| Midfemoral neck fractures | | Treatment | |
|---|---|---|---|
| – Garden 1 | | Conservative | Early functional weight-bearing Loading |
| – Garden 2 | | Conservative/ operative | Screw |
| – Garden 3 | | Operative | Femoral head prosthesis Bipolar prosthesis |
| – Garden 4 | | Operative | Prosthesis |
| Lateral neck fracture Pertrochanteric fracture | | Operative | Dynamic screw and nail and side plate |

## ORTHOPEDIC SURGERY

# Knee

## Knee injuries
### History
The precise mechanism of accident, previous injury, earlier damage, recurrent joint effusion
### Inspection
- External signs of injury, swelling, signs of inflammation, tenderness compared with the other side, alignment of the limb

**Examination** (compare with the other side) Examine the healthy side first

### Tenderness
| | |
|---|---|
| Exterior | lateral meniscus injury, popliteal tendinitis |
| Interior: | medial meniscus injury, varus arthrosis |
| Posterior: | Baker's cyst, popliteal bursitis, ganglion, meniscus |
| Anterior: | irritation of the Hoffa bodies, meniscus injury |
| Course of the lateral ligaments: | lateral ligament injury, tendon insertion disorder |
| Patella: | prepatellar bursitis, patellar chondropathia, effusion joint infection, Sinding–Larsen syndrome, synovitis |
| Femoral condyles: | osteochondrosis, osteochondritis, insertion pathology |
| Tibial tuberosity: | Osgood–Schlatter disease |

**Passive/active movement** (e.g. inhibition of extension by free bodies in the joint or injury to meniscus)
Knee-joint effusion ('dancing' patella), differentiation between intra- and extra-articular injury

### Joint stability
Lachmann test (opening up an anterior cleft on 15° flexion indicates an anterior cruciate ligament rupture)
Posterior movement of the proximal tibia at 90° flexion indicates a posterior cruciate ligament rupture

### Aspiration
Blood-stained fluid indicates fresh trauma, bat globules indicate an intra-articular fracture

### Examination under anesthesia
Manual exam and arthroscopy
Combines diagnosis and treatment

### Relation of passive instability to the ligamentous lesion
[After Muller (1982)]
I   No median opening with isolated lateral/medial ligament rupture on extension, posterior capsule stabilizes the knee joint, opening at 30° flexion is demonstrable
II  Opening on extension indicates cruciate ligament injury
III Lateral opening confirms a cruciate ligament rupture, with questionable associated injury of the iliotibial tract and the popliteal tendon

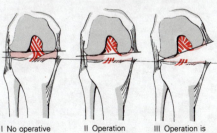

I No operative indication   II Operation is indicated   III Operation is indicated

## MEMORIX SURGERY

## Knee arthroscopy and functional anatomy

**Advantages of arthroscopic operations over arthrotomy**
(From Glintz (1991))
Little postoperative morbidity, shorter period off work, shorter rehabilitation
Outpatient procedure
Hardly any quadriceps inhibition entailed
Better view of the operative site
Less temptation to proceed to unnecessary surgical procedures
Diagnosis and treatment in the same procedure

**Functional anatomy of the knee**

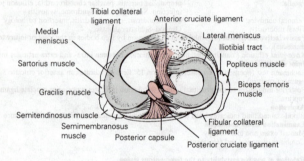

# ORTHOPEDIC SURGERY

## Fractures of the ankle and calcaneus
**Weber's classification of ankle fractures**

|  | Obligatory injury | Facultative associated injury |
|---|---|---|
| Weber A | Fibular fracture distal to intact syndesmosis | Medial ankle fracture |
| Weber B | Fibular fracture at height of syndesmosis | Rupture of anterior syndesmosis, distortion of the posterior Volkmann triangle, medial ankle fracture, rupture of the deltoid ligament |
| Weber C | Fibular fracture proximal to syndesmosis<br>Rupture of syndesmosis<br>Rupture of the interosseous membrane | Distortion of the posterior Volkmann triangle, medial ankle fracture, rupture of the deltoid ligament |

**Maisonneuve fracture:** high Weber C fracture

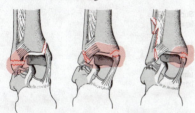

Weber A fracture  Weber B fracture  Weber C fracture

**Tuber–joint angle of the subtalar joint**

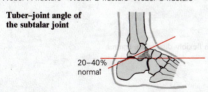

20–40% normal

In fracture of the calcaneus the tuber–joint angle is decreased, with increasing compression

**Operative indications for calcaneal fracture**
- Considerable flattening with decrease of the tuber–joint angle
- Disturbance of the talocalcaneal joint level (CT diagnosis)
- Considerable widening of the heel with fragmentation of the fracture
- Disruption of ligamentary attachments

# MEMORIX SURGERY

## Fractures of the vertebral column

**Three-column principle for the stability of a fractured vertebra**
(After Denis and McAfee)

Anterior column: anterior longitudinal ligament
anterior 2/3 of the vertebral body
annular disc ligaments

Middle column: posterior 1/3 of the vertebral body
annular disc ligaments
posterior longitudinal ligament

Posterior column: vertebral body curvature and its processes
joint capsule
dorsal ligament complex

Anterior, middle, posterior columns

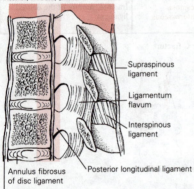

High-grade instability, e.g. from flexion–distraction trauma

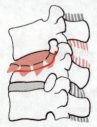

# ORTHOPEDIC SURGERY

## Spinal fractures: diagnosis treatment

### Clinical examination
Pain specification
Particularly in high fractures which are often asymptomatic; here the mechanism of the injury can be a guide

### Radiological examination
X-rays at high, middle, and low levels in two planes
Oblique radiographs to examine the intervertebral foramina and small spinal joints
(Functional radiography – avoid in fresh injury)
CT: examination for a view of the vertebral canal (external method, myelography)
Tomograms
MR
Flexion–extension films

### Treatment
#### Conservative
Traction in the supine position (danger of cord damage, often severe with long-term results)
Bed rest/physiotherapy, exercises
Crutchfield traction
Halo fixation (see figure)
Plaster body jacket (three-point support body jacket)
(see figure)

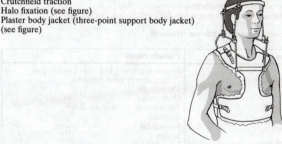

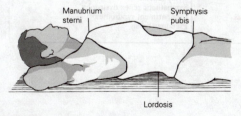

#### Operative
e.g. posterior bone fixation
anterior intervertebral fusion with cancellous grafts

# MEMORIX SURGERY

## Fractures: postoperative care

**Osteosynthesis procedures**
Positional stability (e.g. wire drill fixation)
Stability on exercise (e.g. flat surface bone synthesis)
Partial stability loading (e.g. end nailing, unreamed nail)
weight-bearing stability (e.g. dynamic hip screw)

**Postoperative check**
Position
Bandaging/plaster
Wound
Drainage
Sensation
Muscle strength
Circulation

**Further postoperative treatment**
Isometric exercises (e.g. 'quadriceps training')
Passive motion exercises (e.g. motor splint)
Active motion exercises
Underwater exercises (strengthening exercises)
**Caution:** water resistance increases four-fold with the pace of the exercises

**Complications of operative fracture treatment**

| Symptom | Possible causes |
|---|---|
| Pain | Positioning wrong (e.g. hips hyperflexed, insufficiently erect posture) |
| Swelling | Thrombosis |
| | Overstrain |
| Temperature | Instability of the osteosynthesis |
| | Infection |
| Redness | Hematoma |
| | Serum |
| Immobility | Lymphedema |
| | Sympathetic reflex dystrophy |
| Chronic functional loss | Compartment syndrome |
| Fever | Pseudoarthrosis |
| ESR ↑ leukocytes ↑ | |

# ORTHOPEDIC SURGERY

## Hardware removal

| Hardware removal | Indication | Presumptions for primary fracture healing |
|---|---|---|
| Upper extremity | (+) | Homogeneous bone structure<br>Compact cortical structure<br>Fracture site not visible on plain film |
| Lower extremity | + | |

Table for the optimal timing for the removal of metal implants in fractures assuming an uncomplicated course and proper healing

|  | Min/Max (months) |
|---|---|
| Malleolar fracture (including positioning screw) | 6–12 |
| Tibial shaft | 8–12 |
| Shaft of femur | |
|   plate | 12–18 |
|   medullary nail | 18–24 |
| Head of tibia | 10–18 |
| Patella traction ring | 8–12 |
| Femoral condyles | 12–24 |
| Femoral shaft | |
|   single plate | 24–36 |
|   double plate | From 18 (2 stages) |
|   medullary nail | 24–36 |
| Pertrochanteric/medial neck of femoral fracture | 12–18 |
| Pelvis (only if symptomatic) | From 10 |

**Further indications for metal implant removal**
- Soft tissue problems (redness, infection, perforation)
- Function restriction
- Pain (find the cause)

(From Ruedi and Allgower (1975))

# MEMORIX SURGERY

## Aseptic bone necroses

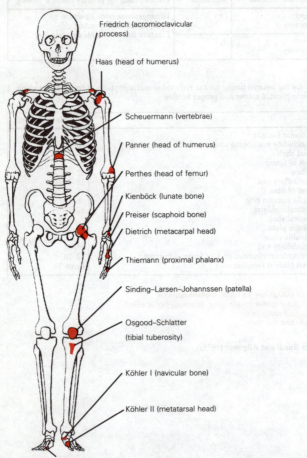

## ORTHOPEDIC SURGERY

## Disorders of locomotion

| Type | Characteristics | Findings |
|---|---|---|
| Short limp | Walks with an up-and-down motion, sheep pelvis, scoliosis | Injured epiphysis |
| Strutting | Deficient joint action is compensated by neighboring joints, multi-positional postures held | Ankylosis<br>Arthrodesis |
| Trendelenberg limp | Waddling gait, unilateral or bilateral: regular steps, Trendelenberg positive; increased lumbar lordosis<br>With slight paresis Duchenne limp | Progressive muscular dystrophy. Girdlestone hip, trochanter major or pseudoarthrosis<br>Gluteal insufficiency, 'congenital' hip dislocation |
| Long-standing limp | Short steps, later pain on walking | Trauma, inflammation<br>Joint affections<br>Femoral head necrosis |
| Cerebellar ataxia | Straddle-legged, irregular, ataxic, list to side | Multiple sclerosis<br>Cerebellar tumor |
| Sensory ataxia | Foot-stamping, four-footed walk or blindfold walking impossible<br>Standing without help impossible | Proprioreceptor loss, cervical retraction, tabes dorsalis, Friedreich ataxia |
| Spastic hemiparesis | Legs held stiffly, circumduction, arms participate | CNS trauma |
| Spastic paraparesis | Both legs strongly adducted (scissor gait)<br>Overcrossing of legs (scissor gait)<br>Cerebral palsy overcrossing of legs, small, regular steps | MS, syringomyelia, spinal<br>Syphilis, cord compression<br>Cerebral paralysis |
| Parkinson gait | Bent forward, short steps, quickening until they fall | Post-encephalitic parkinsonism<br>Phenothiazine treatment<br>Paralysis agitans |
| Extrapyramidal lesions | Athetosis: grotesque distortions, chorea: extreme, varying, accompanying movements<br>Deforming muscular dystonia; spastic<br>Joint contractures (dromedary walk from hip flexion and compensatory lumbar lordosis | Sydenham's chorea<br>Extrapyramidal motor disease, MS |
| Stepping or equine walk (in cauda equina injury) | Paralysis of the foot elevators; forefoot is first drawn up, shoe sole worn in front<br>Legs held abnormally high | Poliomyelitis<br>Peroneal muscle atrophy<br>Charcot-Marie-Tooth<br>Peroneal nerve lesion<br>Tabes dorsalis |
| Drunkard's walk | Staggering, which must be corrected before falling | Intoxication with alcohol, barbiturates |
| Brainstem lesion | Insecurity, sudden unforeseeable stumble and fall | Lateral medulla infarct particularly in the old |
| Hysteric walk | Legs pulled along as superfluous. Dysfunctional walk, normal in bedrest | |
| Frontal lobe lesion | Disequilibrium, feet as stuck together<br>Incapable of balancing, sitting or turning in bed. Cerebral flexion contractures | Tumor, trauma, MS |
| Senile walk | Marche 'à petits pas', short, stiff steps, bent forward | Involution process in frontal lobe and basal ganglia |
| Labyrinthine | Impossible to walk with eyes closed and walk to a fixed point | Streptomycin treatment and aminoglycosides |

(From Holz and Geiselhart (1992))

## Bone tumors

**Classification** (adapted from Atlas of Orthopedic Pathology (1990) Unni, Saunders Publishing)

### 1 Osteoid-forming bone lesions

**Benign**
Osteoid osteoma
Osteoblastoma

**Malignant**
Osteosarcoma (osteogenic sarcoma)
Multicentric osteosarcoma
Low-grade central osteosarcoma
Parosteal osteosarcoma
Periosteal osteosarcoma
Telangiectatic osteosarcoma

### 2 Cartilage-forming bone lesions

**Benign**
Osteochondroma (solitary, multiple, or periosteal)
Chondroma
Chondroblastoma
Chondromyxoid fibroma

**Malignant**
Chondrosarcoma
Chondrosarcoma arising in an osteochondroma
Dedifferentiated chondrosarcoma
Clear cell chondrosarcoma
Mesenchymal chondrosarcoma
Dedifferentiated chondrosarcoma

### 3 Fibrous and fibrohistiocytic lesions

**Benign**
Fibrous dysplasia
Fibroma – metaphyseal fibrous defect
Ossifying fibroma
Benign and atypical fibrous histiocytoma

**Malignant**
Fibrosarcoma
Malignant fibrous histiocytoma

### 4 Hematopoietic lesions

Primary malignant lymphoma
Systemic mastocytosis
Agnogenic myeloid metaplasia (may present as osteosclerotic lesions)

Plasmacytoma and multiple myeloma
Acute leukemia (may present as a lytic lesion)

### 5 Vascular lesions

**Benign**
Hemangioma
Lymphangioma
Hemangiopericytoma

**Malignant**
Malignant hemangiopericytoma
Angiosarcoma

### 6 Miscellaneous bone lesions

Histiocytosis X
Neurilemmoma
Adamantinoma
Giant cell tumor (benign and malignant)
Chordoma

Ewing's sarcoma
Paget's sarcoma
Postradiation sarcoma
Leiomyosarcoma
Lipoma and liposarcoma

### 7 Lesions that may mimic primary bone tumors

Aneurysmal bone cyst
Giant cell reparative granuloma
Hamartoma

Osteofibrous dysplasia
Metastatic carcinoma

### TNM classification of primary malignant bone tumors

(excluding multiple myeloma, juxtacortical osteosarcoma and chondrosarcoma)
T1 limited to the cortex
T2 infiltration through the cortex
N1 regional lymph nodes affected

### Operative indications for palliative treatment

Threatening fracture
Destruction of 50% of the cortex

Diagnostic confirmation
Uncontrollable pain

## ORTHOPEDIC SURGERY

## Compartment syndrome
(see under Nerve compression syndrome (p. 261))

**Definition:** Decreased tissue perfusion through increased interstitial tissue pressure within one or more compartments with consequent neuromuscular disorder and tissue necrosis

**Causes:**
- Trauma: vascular injury, fracture hematoma, soft tissue contusion
- Iatrogenic: enclosed casts or plaster splints or compression bandaging, intra-arterial infusion or transfusion, prolonged intraoperative blood loss, medullary pin osteosynthesis, intramuscular injection, extravasation after intravenous injection or infusion, fascial closure under tension, prolonged elevation of legs, e.g. in hypovolemic shock
- Arterial sclerosis
- Tumor
- Long recumbence after intoxication (e.g. opiates), particularly in the calf

**Diagnosis:**
- Clinically (local pain worsened by pressure, pain in the calf on passive dorsiflexion of the big toe, redness, swelling, induration, contracture)
- Measurement of tissue pressure
- Electromyogram

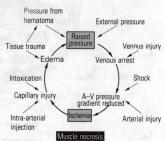

### Clinically important types

| Designation | Compartment affected | Paralyses | Nerve lesions | Specific causes |
|---|---|---|---|---|
| Anterior tibial syndrome | Extensor compartment of lower leg | Anteror tibial, external hallucis longitudinal, external digitorum longus | Deep peroneal nerve | overstretching (football) soft tissue trauma |
| Posterior tibial syndrome | Deep flexion compartment of lower leg | Posterior tibial, flexor hallucis longus, digitorum longus | Tibial nerve | tibial fractures, tibial nailing, venous thrombosis |
| Volkmann's contracture | Flexor compartment of forearm | Deep flexor digitorum, flexor pollicis longus and others | Median nerve and ulnar; rarely radial nerve | ischemia (brachial artery) bleeding faulty injection, ulnar fracture, plaster bandage |

# MEMORIX SURGERY

## Fascial divisions

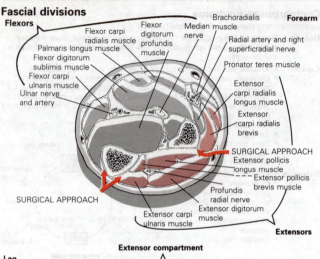

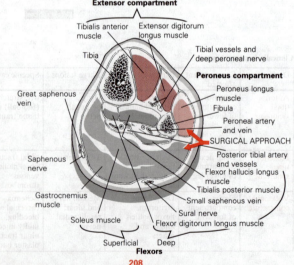

# ORTHOPEDIC SURGERY

## Soft tissue defects and wound closure

**Choice of procedure** depends on:
- Condition of the defect (infection, necrosis)
- Size and position of the defect
- Type of the affected tissue
- Age and condition of the patient
- Other conditions (dexterity of the surgeon, hospital facilities)
- The primary closure (tension-free, no necrosis, no infection)

**Skin grafting**
- Full-thickness, split thickness
- Superficial defects, burns, distant localization
- Technically simple, but depending on a clean vascularized wound bed

**Local/regional flaps**
**Rotation/transposition flaps** (fasciocutaneous)
- Skin/subcutaneous defects
- Often require skin grafting

**Donor sites**
- Technically more difficult, experience necessary

**Axial pattern flap** (fasciocutaneous, myocutaneous)
- Complex defect
- Technically difficult, experience necessary
- Donor site may require skin grafting

**Free microvascular flap** (fasciocutaneous, myocutaneous muscular)
- Complex defects, impaired wound bed
- Technically difficult, experience required

# MEMORIX SURGERY

## Small bone defects
**Treatment; indications**

| Cancellous transplantation | Cortical-cancellous graft transplantation |
|---|---|
| Pathological fracture (after tumor resection<br>Osteoporosis<br>Impression fracture (e.g. head of tibia), compression fracture, cominuted fracture,<br>Delayed healing of fracture<br>Pseudarthrosis (atrophy, defect, necrosis, postinfection)<br>Cyst defect filling<br>Building up socket in the endoprosthesis | Arthrodesis<br>Substitution in osteotomy<br>Lengthening osteotomy |

**Common donor sites**
Anterior iliac crest (a)
Posterior iliac crest (b)
Great trochanter (c)
Head of tibia
Rib
Distal radius
(Proximal ulna)
(Distal tibia)

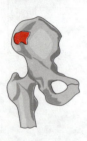
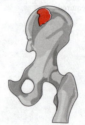
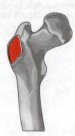

a        b        c

**Possible complications**
Postoperative bleeding
Pain
Nerve injury
Sensory motor disorders
Infection
(Fracture)

## ORTHOPEDIC SURGERY

## Large bone defects
**Corticotomy with callus extraction (after Ilizarov)**
**Indication**:
After radical débridement of avitalized bone and soft tissue fragments
Reconstruction of extensive defects in the long tubular bones
Lengthening of an extremity
Lengthening of an amputation stump
Correction of a defective axial position

**Principle**
To encourage new bone formation after corticotomy (cutting through the cortex protecting the periosteal and medullary blood vessels) with daily extraction of about 1 mm from the corticotomy site

**Free fibula transfer**
Indications:
As above, additionally: the correction of a defective axial position

**Principle:**
Free tissue transfer (bone, fascia, muscle, skin) including microvascular anastomosis

|  | Ilizarov method | Free fibula transfer |
|---|---|---|
| Advantages | More secure method, allows correction of defective axial posture | Shorter duration of treatment |
| Disadvantages | Longer duration of treatment, active cooperation and inspection by the patient required. Difficulty of bone healing in the distal part of the junction | Greater operative effort, wound ridging, possible necrosis of the transplant, operation can only be repeated once |

The psychosocial aspects of an amputation as an alternative should always be considered

## MEMORIX SURGERY

# Amputations and prosthetic care

**Requirements**
Function
Prosthetic capacity
Cosmetic aspect
Earliest possible elimination of pain, to prevent/diminish 'phantom pain' (by plexus or epidural catheter)

## Common amputation levels

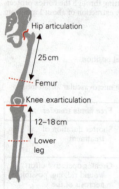

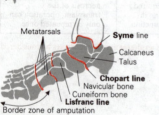

Amputations in the Chopart or Lisfranc lines are unsatisfactory because of the resulting imbalance between flexors and extensors. A valid alternative is the tenodesis or arthrodesis of the ankle.

**Prosthetic care**
Considerations are:
The amputation level
Amputation technique
**Weight-bearing capacity of the stump (myoplastic or osteoplastic**
except knee exarticulation)
Earliest possible provision of the prosthesis
Training in the use of the limb substitute

# HAND SURGERY

## Replantation

**Transportation of an amputated part**

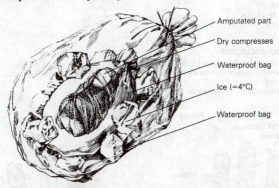

- Amputated part
- Dry compresses
- Waterproof bag
- Ice (=4°C)
- Waterproof bag

**Considerations for replantation**
- The pre-existing disability, age, occupation, important leisure-time activity, sex
- The predicted functional loss without replantation
- The anticipated function of the replanted part after replantation

| Absolute indications | Relative indications | No indication |
| --- | --- | --- |
| Thumb<br>Multiple digits<br>Hand, ear, scalp, foot, penis | Distal digit amputations<br>Single digits<br>Crush/avulsion injuries<br>Leg | Life-threatening injury<br>Pre-existing medical condition<br>Poor condition of amputated part |

**Normal sequence of operative procedures during replantation**
1. Fracture reduction and fixation
2. Tendon repair
3. Arterial anastomosis  ⎫ may vary
4. Venous anastomosis  ⎭
5. Nerve repair

# MEMORIX SURGERY

## Anesthesia

**Types of anesthetic**
- Digital block
- Bier block
- Axillary block ●●
- General ••

## Common incisions

- Creases should not be crossed at 90° angles
- Skin flexion/extension creases should not be crossed at a 90° angle unless Z-plasties are planned
- Subcutaneous veins on the dorsal hand should be preserved

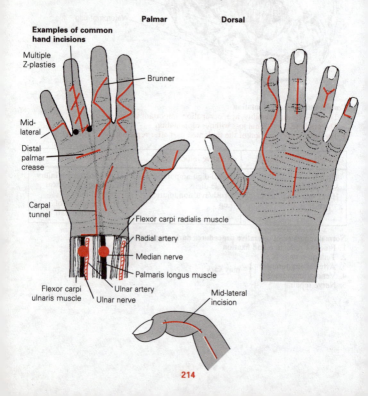

# HAND SURGERY

## Relaxation position

**Relaxation position** (for best future mobilization)
- Wrist joint: 30–40° extension
- MCP joint: 90° flexion
- PIP joint: 0° flexion
- DIP joint: 0° flexion

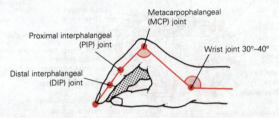

**Dynamic splinting used after flexor tendon repair** (after Kleinert)
- Repaired finger held in flexion by a rubber band which allows active extension to a dorsal blocking splint
- Passive motion of repaired flexor tendon allows healing without adhesions
- Traction on finger directed toward the scaphoid
- Traction on thumb directed toward the fifth metacarpal head

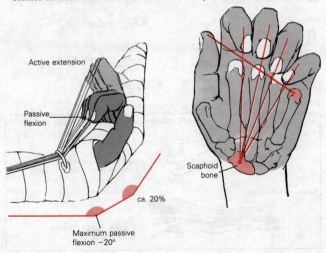

## MEMORIX SURGERY

## Tendons and tendon injuries
### Cross-section proximal to the wrist joint

- Flexor carpi radialis muscle
- Median nerve
- Radius
- Radial artery
- Palmaris long tendon
- Ulnar artery
- Ulnar nerve

**I–VI** Extensor tendon compartments (I–VI)

- **I** Abductor pollicis longus muscle; Extensor pollicis brevis muscle
- **II** Extensor carpi radialis longus muscle; Extensor carpi radialis brevis muscle
- **III** Extensor pollicis longus muscle
- **IV** Extensor digitorum communis muscle; Extensor indicis proprius muscle
- **V** Extensor digiti minimi muscle
- **VI** Extensor carpi ulnaris muscle

- Flexis pollicis longus
- Flexor carpi ulnaris tendon
- Flexor digitorum profundis tendons
- Ulnar styloid process

Tendon suture modif. Kirchmair (Kessler)

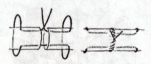

Pulvertaft's weave (secondary reconstruction, tendon graft)

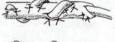

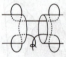

External tendon imbalance

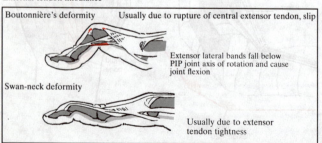

Boutonnière's deformity — Usually due to rupture of central extensor tendon, slip

Extensor lateral bands fall below PIP joint axis of rotation and cause joint flexion

Swan-neck deformity

Usually due to extensor tendon tightness

# HAND SURGERY

## Chronic diseases of the hand

**Dupuytren's contraction**
- Unknown etiology, palmar fibroblast proliferation of collagen and contracture of palmar aponeurosis
- Operative indication: pain, decreased digital extension
- Treatment:
  - Partial palmar fasciectomy, selective cord excision, or transection
  - Z-plasty or local flap may be required for the closure

**Tenosynovitis (inflammation of the tendon sheath)**
- Multiple etiology (e.g. congenital, chronic inflammatory, repeated steroid injection)
- **deQuervains'' tenosynovitis**
  - Affects the first extensor tendon compartment
  - Diagnosis by positive Finkelstein test (pain with ulnar deviation of the thumb)
  - Treatment: release of the tendon compartment

Caution: the superficial portion of the median nerve may easily be injured.

**Trigger finger**
- Constriction of flexor tendon sheath at A1 pulley in palm or flexor tendon swelling
- Diagnosis: snapping of the digit into the palm during full range of active flexion and when extending
- Treatment
- Division of the A1 pulley

Caution: injury to digital neurovascular bundles

**Arthritis**
Etiology: joint surface degeneration
Symptoms: morning stiffness, swelling, pain, distorted joint contour; radiologically: sclerosis of joint surfaces, subchondral cyst formation
The clinical symptoms and radiological findings do not necessarily correspond
Treatment:
- Conservative (medical)
- Denervation
- Arthroplasty
- Synthetic joint replacement
- Arthrodesis (joint fusion)

The most common joint affected is the basilar thumb joint

**Tendonopathy/tenosynovitis**
- Inflammatory, degenerative
- Under/overloading syndrome with pain in the region of the tendon attachment and tendon sheath
- Treatment
  - Conservative (physiotherapy, rest)
  - Denervation
  - Synovectomy
  - Disinsertion of the relevant musculature

**Rheumatism**
- Inflammatory, autoimmune, unknown
- Swelling, pain, decreased hand function, joint destruction from proliferative synovitis (classically: ulnar deviation of hand)
- Treatment: conservative, early synovectomy, joint replacement, arthrodesis

## MEMORIX SURGERY

## Infections of the hand

### Symptoms
Typical inflammatory signs (cellulitis treatment)
Kanavel's sign – ref: tenosynovitis (purulence in digital flexor tendon sheath)
1. Finger held in flexion
2. Swelling of finger
3. Pain in palpation along the course of the tendon sheath
4. Pain on passive finger extension

Rx: surgical drainage of tendon sheath

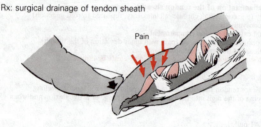

### Infection: can migrate proximally along tendon sheaths

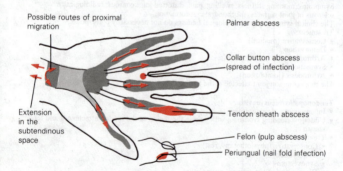

- Possible routes of proximal migration
- Extension in the subtendinous space
- Palmar abscess
- Collar button abscess (spread of infection)
- Tendon sheath abscess
- Felon (pulp abscess)
- Periungual (nail fold infection)

### Treatment
**Pyogenic infection is an indication for operative intervention**
- Incision
- Necrectomy
- Drainage
- Antibiotics
- Débridement
- Irrigation
- Elevation
- Immobilization

Caution: palm abscess can spread dorsally

# HAND SURGERY

## Wound closure of hand defects

**1**
- Split thickness skin graft
- Full thickness skin graft

**2 Local – regional**
- V–Y flap (Tranquilli–Leali, Attasoy; volar advancement flap)
  (Kutler: bilateral advancement flap)
- Cross-finger flap
- Transposition flap covering the adjacent defect
- pedicled forearm flap (radial, ulnar) with flow reversal through palmar arch

**3 Distant flap**
- Groin flap
- Chest wall/cross-arm flap

**4 Free tissue transfer with microvascular anastomoses**
- Skin flap (scapular, parascapular, deltoid, lateral arm, forearm)
- Muscle flap (latissimus dorsi, serratus, rectus abdominis)
- Fascial flap/STSG (temporalis, parascapular, deltoid, scapular)
- Skin–muscle flap (latissimus, rectus abdominis)

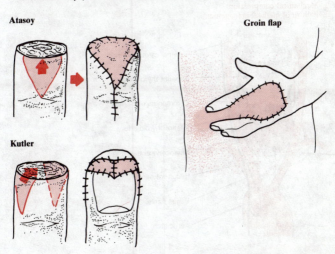

Atasoy

Kutler

Groin flap

219

## MEMORIX SURGERY

**Diagnostic studies**
1. Thyroid scan – $^{99m}$Tc (nuclear medicine)
   a) Hot nodule – hyperfunction, cancer unlikely
   b) Cold nodule – more suspicious for cancer but only 20–30% of cold nodules will contain cancer
2. Fine-needle aspiration
   a) 'Gold' standard for diagnosing thyroid nodules
   b) False positives rare – false negatives more common
   c) Requires good pathologist for reliable results
3. Ultrasound – differentiates cold from cystic nodules; rarely indicated

**Preoperative evaluation**
1. Careful H & P – if family history, hyperparathyroidism, or hypertension, consider MEN syndrome
2. Chest X-ray – rule out substernal goiter or pulmonary mets
3. Labs – CBC, UA, chemistry profile, TSH
4. Indirect laryngoscopy – to evaluate vocal cord function, especially if hoarseness present

**Operative indications**
1. Suspicion of malignancy
2. Mechanical compression
3. Failure of medical management

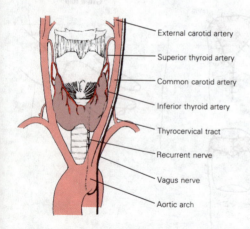

External carotid artery
Superior thyroid artery
Common carotid artery
Inferior thyroid artery
Thyrocervical tract
Recurrent nerve
Vagus nerve
Aortic arch

# ENDOCRINE SURGERY

## Thyroid
### Classification
Two general categories of surgically treated thyroid disease:
1. Thyroid nodule/carcinoma
2. Hyperthyroidism

### Evaluation of thyroid nodule
- Most patients clinically euthyroid
- Differential diagnosis
  1. Benign:
     a) follicular adenoma – most common benign thyroid nodule; 85%
     b) thyroid cysts
     c) nodular goiter
  2. Malignant (see Table)
     a) papillary – well-differentiated, best prognosis
     b) follicular – well-differentiated, good prognosis
     c) medullary – associated with MEN syndrome
        - multicentric; elevated calcitonin
     d) anaplastic – poorly differentiated, worst prognosis
     e) other – lymphoma
        - tall cell variant of papillary Ca. – rare, much worse prognosis, overall mortality 30%, uniformly fatal if metastatic at diagnosis

### Characteristics of thyroid carcinoma
(From Rothmund (1990))

| Carcinoma | Papillary | Follicular | Medullary | Anaplastic |
|---|---|---|---|---|
| Frequency (%) | 65 | 25 | 5 | 5 |
| Proportion of females (%) | 70 | 70 | 55 | 60 |
| Mortality from ca. (% age of all patients) | 5 | 25 | 35 | 98 |
| Metastases | | | | |
| lymphogenic | +++ | + | +++ | ++ |
| hematogenic | + | +++ | + | +++ |
| Iodine take-up | ++ | +++ | – | – |
| Grade of malignancy | + | ++ | +++ | extreme |

# Hyperparathyroidism

## Operative technique
1. Transverse cervical incision, elevation of subplatysmal flap, separation of strap muscles (sternothyroid sternohyoid thyrohyoid) in midline
2. Identify recurrent laryngeal nerve located in triangle bounded by the inferior thyroid artery, trachea, and carotid artery
3. Preserve parathyroid glands
4. Ligate the superior thyroid artery
5. Rotate thyroid lobe medially and detach Berry's suspensory ligament to release the thyroid lobe from the trachea.

- The minimum operation is lobectomy and isthmusectomy
- Most surgeons agree that if carcinoma is present, a total thyroidectomy is indicated due to multicentricity and low incidence of complications, i.e. recurrent nerve injury and hypoparathyroidism
- Generally treat postoperatively with $^{131}$I radiation

## Evaluation of hyperthyroidism
- H & P – heat intolerance, palpitations, sweating, weight loss, tachycardia
- Classification a) Grave's disease – diffuse toxic goiter
  b) Plummer's disease – solitary toxic nodule
- Thyroid function tests:
  a) TSH – level high if etiology of hyperthyroidism is pituitary adenoma
  – level low if etiology of hyperthyroidism is thyroid due to negative feedback
  b) $T_4$ – half-life 7 days (firmly bound to plasma protein)
  c) $T_3$ – half-life 3 days

## Treatment
Generally treat hyperthyroidism with:
1. $^{131}$I radiation – dose depends on the size of the gland, generally 10–30 mCi
2. Antithyroid medications:
   - propylthiouracil 150 mg p.o. q8h
   - methimazole 10 mg p.o. q8h
   - side effect – agranulocytosis

## Indications for surgical treatment of hyperthyroidism
1. Pregnant females with hyperthyroidism who cannot be controlled with low doses of antithyroid medication
2. Patients intolerant of radiation or medical therapy

Preoperative treatment for hyperthyroidism
1. Establish euthyroid state with antithyroid medications
2. β-blockers to prevent cardiac tachyarrhythmias
3. Consider iodine solutions (Lugol's, SSKI) for negative feedback effect.

Operative treatment is subtotal thyroidectomy

# ENDOCRINE SURGERY

## APUD system

### The APUD system: Amine Precursor Uptake and Decarboxylation
- Taking up amines and their precursors, decarboxylation, formation of different polypeptides
- Origin from neural crest (ectoderm)
- Inheritance – sporadic 85–90%
  – autosomal dominant 10–15%

### MEN syndromes

| | |
|---|---|
| MEN I | • parathyroid hyperplasia<br>• pancreatic islet cell neoplasms<br>• pituitary neoplasms |
| MEN IIA | • medullary thyroid carcinoma<br>• pheochromocytoma<br>• parathyroid hyperplasia |
| MEN IIB | • medullary thyroid carcinoma<br>• pheochromocytoma<br>• mucosal neuromas |

### Pituitary tumors
- Mostly benign adenomas of the anterior lobe
- Hypersecretion from a hormone-producing tumor
- Insufficient hormone production from tumor compression

**Diagnosis:** radiography of sella turcica, slice pictures of the sella, CT, NMR
**Treatment:** excision, trans-sphenoidal hypophysectomy

| Hormone | Clinical picture |
|---|---|
| Growth hormone (GH) | Acromegaly |
| Prolactin (PRI) | Galactorrhea |
| Melanocyte-stimulating hormone (MSH) | Pigmentation |
| Thyrotropic hormone (TSH) | Hyperthyroidism |
| Adrenocorticotrophic hormone (ACTH) | Hypercortisonism |

223

# Pheochromocytoma and endocrine pancreatic tumors

**Pheochromocytoma**
Secretes epinephrine and norepinephrine
**Symptoms** – hypertension, tachycardia, perspiration, weight loss, facial pallor, headache

### Diagnosis
1. 24-hour urinary excretion of catecholamines and vanillylmandelic acid; most sensitive and specific test
2. Plasma catecholamines
3. CT scan abdomen – to localize the tumor, 10% bilateral, 10% extra-adrenal
Most common location of extra-adrenal pheochromocytoma is at the aortic bifurcation called the Organ of Zuckerkandl

**Preoperative treatment** – adrenergic blockade with pheoxybenzamine or phentolamine

### Operative treatment
1. Midline laparotomy
2. Ligate adrenal vein early to prevent catecholamines from entering the systemic circulation during manipulation of the tumor

### Endocrine pancreatic tumors

| Tumor | Cells | Hormone secretion |
|---|---|---|
| Glucagonoma | A | Glucagon |
| Insulinoma | B | Insulin |
| Somatostatinoma | D | Somatostatin |
| Gastrinoma | G | Gastrin |
| PP-oma | PP | Pancreatic polypeptides |
| Vipoma | $D_1$ | Vasoactive intestinal polypeptides |
| Carcinoid | EC | Serotonin |

### Carcinoid
- Generally slow-growing
- Metastases to lymphatics and liver
- Secretes serotonin (5HT)

### Symptoms
Flushing, colicky abdominal pain (carcinoid syndrome) – generally systemic effects of carcinoid tumors in GI tract are only apparent after metastasis since the first-pass effect metabolizes serotonin before entry into the systemic circulation

### Diagnosis
↑ 5-Hydroxyindole acetic acid in 24-hour urine collections

### Anatomic
Location – appendix 45%, ileum 30%, rectum 15%

### Operative treatment
- Appendiceal carcinoid – appendectomy if tumor <2 cm; right colectomy if tumor >2 cm
- Rectal carcinoid – wide local excision, APR only for salvage
- Small bowel carcinoid – segmental small bowel resection

# ENDOCRINE SURGERY

## Gastrinoma

*Zollinger–Ellison syndrome (gastrinoma)*
Frequency <1% of all ulcer patients
Classic triad – gastric hypersecretion, recurrent peptic ulceration, resistant to medical treatment
Symptoms – abdominal pain, ↑ gastric acid secretion, vomiting, diarrhea
Diagnosis – elevated serum gastrin >400 pg/ml is diagnostic
– secretin stimulation test: 2 mg/kg i.v. – if gastrin level increases more than 200 pg/ml diagnosis is positive

**Location** – most tumors (85%) found in gastrinoma triangle, which is the area bounded by the neck of the pancreas, the junction of the second and third portions of the duodenum, and the junction of the cystic and common bile duct. May localize with CT scan or selective angiography.

**Treatment**
Conservative – cimetidine
– $H_2$ blockers cimetidine, ranitidine
– omeprazole
Operative – explore for resection of gastrinoma
– total gastrectomy as a salvage procedure

**Differential diagnosis of hypergastrinemia**
Antral G-cell hyperplasia
Retained antrum after incomplete antrectomy
Pernicious anemia
Chronic renal insufficiency
Gastrinoma

## Paraneoplastic syndromes

ACTH: carcinoid, colon, liver, lungs, breast, adrenal, pancreas, uterus
Erythropoietin: hemangioblastoma
FSH: lungs
Gastrin: lungs, stomach
Glucagon: lungs, stomach
HCG: choriocarcinoma, germ cell tumor, lungs
Insulin: lungs
Calcitonin: lungs, breast, stomach, thyroid
LH: liver, lungs
Parathormone: endometrium, lungs, breast, kidneys, esophagus, ovary, vulva, cervix
TSH: lungs, breast

## MEMORIX SURGERY

## Investigations
**Palpation and auscultation of the arterial vascular system**
(Modified from Haring, R. and Zilch, H. (1986))

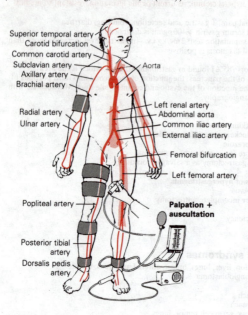

- Superior temporal artery
- Carotid bifurcation
- Common carotid artery
- Subclavian artery
- Axillary artery
- Brachial artery
- Aorta
- Radial artery
- Ulnar artery
- Left renal artery
- Abdominal aorta
- Common iliac artery
- External iliac artery
- Femoral bifurcation
- Left femoral artery
- Popliteal artery
- Posterior tibial artery
- Dorsalis pedis artery

**Palpation + auscultation**

**Cardiac auscultation is mandatory**

**Pressure indices**

$$\text{Ankle–brachial index (ABI)} = \frac{\text{Systolic pressure in the posterior tibial or dorsalis pedis arteries}}{\text{Systolic pressure in the brachial artery}}$$

Analogues for calculation of the more distal segmental pressure indices (see figure)
- below the knee
- above the knee
- proximal thigh

**Predication**
>1: normal
>0.5: single occlusion
<0.5: multiple occlusions

**Progress check:**
Descending index = worsening of the disease
Ascending index = formation of collaterals

# VASCULAR SURGERY AND THE LYMPHATIC SYSTEM

## Classification of arterial aneurysms

**Morphology**
True aneurysm
- sack (a)
- fusiform (b)
- dissecting (c)

False aneurysm (d)
(= false artery, 'pulsating hematoma')

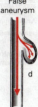

Venous aneurysm fusiform, sacciform — Dissecting aneurysm — False aneurysm

**Etiology**
- congenital
- arteriosclerotic
- mycotic
- traumatic
- syphilitic

**Clinically**
closed
- asymptomatic
- symptomatic

ruptured

**Situation**
- peripheral
- central

**De Bakey classification of dissecting aortic aneurysms**
I  Dissection of the ascending to the descending aorta
II Dissection restricted to ascending aorta
III Dissection beginning distal to left subclavian artery

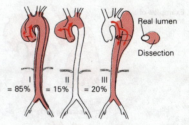

= 85%  = 15%  = 20%

Real lumen

Dissection

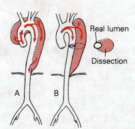

Real lumen

Dissection

**Stanford classification of aortic dissection**
A Dissection includes the ascending aorta and aortic arch
B Dissection does not include the ascending aorta

# MEMORIX SURGERY

## Diagnosis and treatment of arterial aneurysms

**Diagnostic aids**
- Sonography
- Computed tomography
- Angiography (only if surgery is anticipated)

**Diagnosis and treatment of infrarenal aortic aneurysms**
(From Dorrler and Hoffman (1989))

**Abdominal aortic aneurysms (AA)**

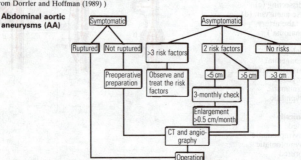

**Examples of surgical treatment**

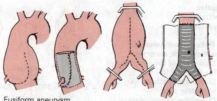

Fusiform aneurysm of ascending aorta

Infrarenal aortic aneurysm

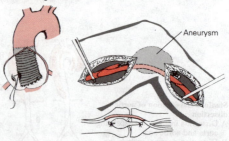

Popliteal aneurysm

## VASCULAR SURGERY AND THE LYMPHATIC SYSTEM

### Cerebral ischemia
**Severity of cerebral ischemia and its relation to operative indication**
(From Hamann and Volmar (1989))

| Severity | | Pattern of symptoms | Surgical indications |
|---|---|---|---|
| Stage I | | Asymptomatic stenosis | + |
| Stage II<br>TIA (transient ischemic attack), intermittent cerebrovascular insufficiency; 'impending stroke', 'little stroke', angiospastic insult; TRINS (total reversible ischemic neurological symptoms) | | Frequent recurrence of attacks: duration of neurological symptoms: minutes to 24 h with complete resolution | +++ |
| Stage III<br>Acute apoplectic stroke, cerebral infarct; 'acute stroke', 'progressive stroke'; PRIND (prolonged ischemic neurological deficit) TRINS (total reversible ischemic symptoms) | >24 h | Ischemic insult: lasting longer than 24 h but with clinical resolution | (+)<br>Up to 6–8 h of unconsciousness |
| | >24 h | Ischemic insult | |
| PRINS (partial reversible ischemic neurological symptoms) | | | |
| Stage IV<br>Post-apoplectic condition: 'completed stroke'. IRINS (irreversible ischemic neurological symptoms | or | Permanent neurological symptoms after 4 weeks 'Partial defect' partial remission possible | (+)<br>Correction of contralateral stenosis |

229

## Carotid stenosis

**Doppler sonographic criteria in the quantification of carotid stenosis**
(After Hennerici and Neuerburg-Heusler (1988))

| | Non-stenotic plaque | Minimum stenosis | Medium stenosis | High-grade stenosis | Subtotal stenosis | Closure |
|---|---|---|---|---|---|---|
| Lumen narrowing | <40% | 40–60% | 60–70% | >80% | >90% | 100% |
| Indirect criteria | None | None | None | Supraorbital blood flow, retrograde common carotid flow diminution in side-to-side comparison | | |
| **Direct criteria in the stenosis area:** | | | | | | |
| Continuous Doppler | None | Abruptly increased blood flow | Distinct flow increase Pulsatile loss, systolic deceleration (turbulence) | Strong increase, systolic deceleration | Variable stenosis signal with lower intensity | Absent vessels |
| Frequency-time spectrum | None | Spread | Spread, increased low-frequency part | Reduced, inverse frequency | Reduced, inverse frequency | Absent vessels |
| Post-stenotic findings | None | None | None | Diminished systolic flow velocity | Reduced, signal difficult | Absent signal |
| Systolic peak frequency of internal carotid artery (with 4 MHz transmission frequency) | <3 kHz | 3–5 kHz | 5–8 kHz | >8 kHz | Variable | Absent |
| Diagnosis in B-mode technique | Very good | Very good | Good | Moderate | Moderate | Poor |

# VASCULAR SURGERY AND THE LYMPHATIC SYSTEM

## Arterial obstruction

**History in arterial closure**
**Onset:**
- sudden: embolism
- slow: thrombosis

**Causes: arteriosclerosis** (>90%), inflammatory, vascular disease, external compression, cysts, adventitial degeneration, fibromuscular dysplasia, stenosis (congenital, acquired)

*Risk factors*: smoking, hypertension, fat metabolism disorders, diabetes mellitus, hyperglobulinemia, polycythemia, thrombocytosis

**Symptoms**: exercise-dependent, free intervals, intermittent claudication, pain on walking, pain increased on foot elevation, pain at rest

**Classification of peripheral arterial obstruction** (Fontaine)

| Stage | Criteria for staging | Sub-grouping (walking) | Ankle arterial pressure (in normotensives) (Marshall) | Ankle–brachial index | Operative indication |
|---|---|---|---|---|---|
| I | Objective disease, no subjective symptoms | | 100 mmHg | 0.9–0.75 | |
| II | Intermittent claudication | IIa Pain-free walking over 100–200 m<br>IIb pain-free walking under 100–200 m | 90–60 mmHg | 0.75–0.5 | (+) |
| III | Pain at rest | | ≤50 mmHg | <0.5 | + |
| IV | Necrosis (gangrene) | | ≤50 mmHg | <0.5 | + |

Medial calcification can give falsely elevated pressures.

Ankle arterial pressures over 160–180 mmHg in normotensives suggest medial calcification, sclerosis or edema. Values above 300 mmHg indicate medial calcification or aortic insufficiency.

## *MEMORIX SURGERY*

## Arteries of the pelvis

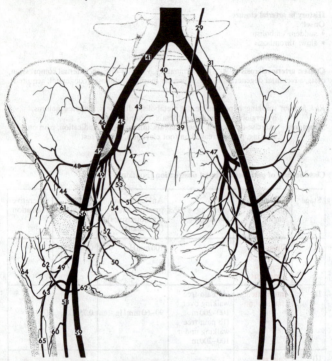

- 40 Middle sacral artery
- **41 Common iliac artery**
- **42 External iliac artery**
- 43 Inferior epigastric artery
- 44 Deep circumflex artery
- 45 Internal iliac artery (hypogastric artery)
- 46 Iliolumbar artery
- 47 Lateral sacral artery
- 48 Superior gluteal artery
- 49 Inferior gluteal artery
- 50 Internal pudendal artery
- 51 Middle rectal artery
- 52 Obturator artery
- 53 Uterine artery
- 54 Inferior vesical artery
- 55 Superficial epigastric artery
- **56 Common femoral artery**
- 57 External pudendal artery
- **58 Deep femoral artery**
- **59 Superficial femoral artery**
- 60 Perforating arteries
- 61 Superficial circumflex iliac artery
- 62 Medial femoral circumflex artery (tibial)
- 63 Lateral femoral circumflex artery (fibular)
- 64 Ascending ramus of lateral circumflex femoris artery
- 65 Descending ramus of lateral circumflex femoris artery

(From Muller *et al.*)

# VASCULAR SURGERY AND THE LYMPHATIC SYSTEM

## Arteries of the leg

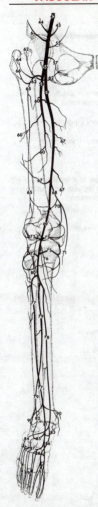

42 **External iliac artery**
43 Inferior epigastric artery
44 Deep circumflex iliac artery
45 Internal iliac artery (hypogastric artery)
46 Iliolumbar artery
47 Lateral sacral artery
48 Superior gluteal artery
49 Inferior gluteal artery
50 Internal pudendal artery
51 Middle rectal artery
52 Obturator artery
53 Uterine artery
54 Inferior vesical artery
55 Superficial epigastric artery
56 **Common femoral artery**
57 External pudendal artery
58 **Deep femoral artery**
59 **Superficial femoral artery**
60 Perforating arteries
61 Superficial circumflex iliac artery
62 Middle femoral circumflex artery (tibial)
63 Lateral femoral circumflex artery (fibular)
64 Ascending branch of lateral femoral circumflex artery
65 Descending ramus of lateral femoral circumflex artery
66 Transverse branch of lateral femoral circumflex artery
67 Muscle branches of femoral and deep femoral arteries
68 Descending genicular artery
69 **Popliteal artery**
70 Articular branch of descending genicular artery
71 Saphenous branch of descending genicular artery
72 Superior lateral genicular artery
73 Superior medial genicular artery
74 Inferior lateral genicular artery
75 Inferior medial genicular artery
76 Sural artery
77 **Anterior tibial artery**
78 **Posterior tibial artery**
79 **Peroneal artery (fibular artery)**
80 Anterior tibial recurrent artery
81 **Dorsalis pedis artery**
82 Perforating branch of peroneal artery
83 Internal tarsal artery
84 Lateral plantaris artery
85 Lateral tarsal artery
86 Medial plantaris artery
87 Arcuate artery
88 Deep branch of dorsalis pedis artery
89 Dorsal metatarsal, plantar metatarsal, dorsal and plantar digital artery
90 Anterior medial malleolar artery
91 Anterior lateral malleolar artery

(From Muller *et al.*)

# MEMORIX SURGERY

## Surgical treatment of vascular block

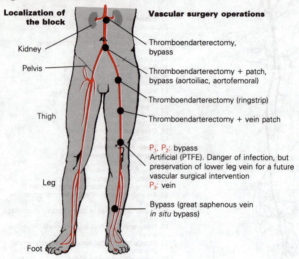

**Localization of the block**: Kidney, Pelvis, Thigh, Leg, Foot

**Vascular surgery operations**:
- Thromboendarterectomy, bypass
- Thromboendarterectomy + patch, bypass (aortoiliac, aortofemoral)
- Thromboendarterectomy (ringstrip)
- Thromboendarterectomy + vein patch
- $P_1$, $P_2$: bypass
  Artificial (PTFE). Danger of infection, but preservation of lower leg vein for a future vascular surgical intervention
  $P_3$: vein
- Bypass (great saphenous vein *in situ* bypass)

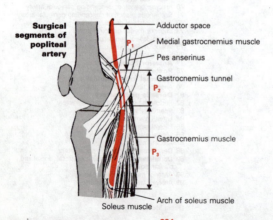

**Surgical segments of popliteal artery**
- Adductor space
- Medial gastrocnemius muscle
- Pes anserinus
- Gastrocnemius tunnel
- Gastrocnemius muscle
- Arch of soleus muscle
- Soleus muscle

# VASCULAR SURGERY AND THE LYMPHATIC SYSTEM

## Acute peripheral arterial block
### Symptoms

| Pratt's 6 'P's' | Pain<br>Paresthesia<br>Paralysis<br>Pallor<br>Pulselessness<br>Prostration |
|---|---|

### Etiology
### Arterial embolus
Cardiac – Cause in 80–90% of all arterial emboli (coronary heart disease, myocardial aneurysm, valvular disease, artificial valve, endocarditis)
Aneurysms (aortic, periarticular arteries, e.g. popliteal)
Ulcerated arteriosclerotic plaque, tumor fragments, fat, air, foreign body
Paradoxical embolus (pelvic, lung, leg thrombus through a patent foramen ovale)

### Arterial thrombosis
Closure of an arteriosclerotic plaque, cystic adventitial degeneration

### Traumatic
Fracture, dislocation (intimal lesion)
Compression (hematoma, 'entrapment', compartmental syndrome)

### Iatrogenic
Vascular puncture, dilatation, reconstruction
Accidental injection (barbiturates, tranquilizers, synthetic penicillin, sclerosing preparations)

### Ergotism
Methysergine-containing preparations, ergotamine-containing heparin

### Aortic dissection with obstruction of lumen

### Phlegmasia cerulea dolens

# MEMORIX SURGERY

## Acute peripheral arterial obstruction

**Diagnostic and therapeutic procedures in arterial block of the extremities**
(From Zuhlke *et al.* (1990))

IOTA – intraoperative transluminal angioplasty; PTA – percutaneous transluminal angioplasty; PTEE – percutaneous thromboembolectomy

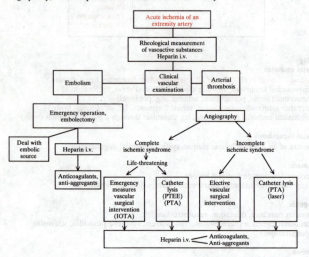

## Differential diagnosis
(Modified from Dembrowski (1959))

| Symptoms | Arterial embolism | Arterial thrombosis | Phlegmasia cerulea dolena | Traumatic injury | Dissecting aneurysm |
|---|---|---|---|---|---|
| History | Heart disease, atrial fibrillation, infarct | Arteriosclerosis, local injury | Recurrent thrombophlebitis | Vascular trauma | Hypertension pregnancy Lax connective tissue (Marfan's syndrome) |
| Onset | Acute | Acute to subacute | Acute to subacute | Acute | Acute |
| Pain | Severe | Moderately severe | Moderately severe | Severe | Moderate |
| Skin color | Pale | Pale | Cyanotic | Pale | Pale |
| Edema | None | None | Present | None | None |
| Skin veins | Collapsed | Collapsed | Distended | Collapsed | (Collapsed?) |
| Pulse | Weak | Weak | Weak | Weak | Changing |
| Skin | Cold | Cold | Normal | Cold | Cold |
| Arteriogram | Cupola, flat | Degenerative changes | Narrowed | Narrowed | Double contour |

# VASCULAR SURGERY AND THE LYMPHATIC SYSTEM

## Vascular surgery: techniques
- Transverse incision → primary closure (1)
- Longitudinal incision → patch plasty (2)
- Thromboendarterectomy (TEA) (3)
- Bypass (anatomic 4, extra-anatomic 5)
- Percutaneous transluminal angioplasty
- (Rotation endarterectomy)
- Insertion of intraluminal stents
- Laser dispersion of stenosis

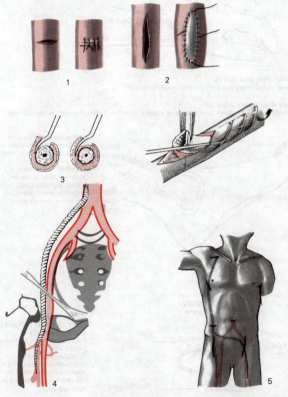

## Dialysis shunts

### Requirements
Adequate arterial flow
Small shunt volume (cardiac effort)
Minimal ischemic danger for the affected extremity
Good access
Good functional capacity, low complication rate

### Cimino shunt
Subcutaneous fistula between artery and neighboring vein. Arterializing of the vein, usually by end-to-side anastomosis (see figure)

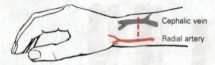

Indication: long-term dialysis
Location: radial artery and cephalic vein (wrist, forearm)

### Scribner shunt (rarely indicated)
Extracorporeal plastic shunt, interposition of a plastic tube (i.e. Teflon) between artery and vein

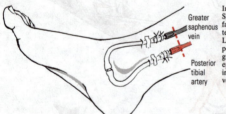

Indication: hemofiltration. Short-term dialysis, acute renal failure, initial phase of long-term dialysis
Location: radial artery and vein, posterior tibial artery and greater saphenous vein (inferior epigastric artery and vein), internal mammary artery and vein

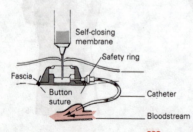

### Atrial catheter
Shunt method (e.g. Demers or Quinton catheter)
Location: external or internal jugular vein (1) or (3). Conduction through a subcutaneous tunnel with a subcutaneous bacterial filter, the catheter tip is placed in the right atrium

# VASCULAR SURGERY AND THE LYMPHATIC SYSTEM

## Deep pelvic and femoral venous thrombosis

### Symptoms and diagnosis
**Problems**
- Danger of pulmonary embolism
- Danger of recurrent thrombosis
- Danger of development of a post-thrombotic syndrome

**Risk factors**
- Stasis (postoperative immobilization, immobilizing bandaging, prolonged sitting, paralysis of the extremities)
- Local vascular damage (intravenous catheter, trauma, burns)
- Hypercoagulability (low AT-III, hormonal dysfunction, ovulation inhibitors, estrogens, malignancy)
- Others (age over 40, previous phlebitis, pregnancy, obesity, family predisposition)

**Clinical symptoms**
- Pale, shiny, livid or cyanotic skin color
- Tenderness in the course of the deep veins
- Projection of superficial veins
- Ankle edema
- Light pain, better when lying down
- Feeling ill
- Nonspecific complaints

**Diagnostic aids**
- Phlebography (for diagnosis and follow-up)
- Duplex sonography
- Doppler sonography
- Plethysmography

**Venous ultrasound Doppler signals at the groin**
(From Martin, M. and Fiebach, B.J.O. (1988))

| | | |
|---|---|---|
| A | Normal respiration, venous current signal over the groin | A Current signal in a healthy subject at rest |
| B | Normal respiration with deep inspiration, venous current signal over the groin | B On deep inspiration the current signal disappears as a sign of patency of the pelvic veins |
| C | Normal respiration with deep inspiration, venous current signal over the groin | C No disappearance of the venous current signal on deeper inspiration is a sign of pelvic flow obstruction |
| D | Normal respiration, venous current signal over the groin<br><br>Manual pressure on the abdomen | D On light manual pressure on the abdomen in a healthy subject the venous current signal over the groin disappears |
| E | Normal respiration, venous current signal over the groin<br><br>Manual pressure on the abdomen | E In a patient with iliac vein thrombosis the venous current signal over the groin disappears in spite of manual compression of the abdomen |

# MEMORIX SURGERY

**Treatment**
**General treatment**
- Acute stage – *elevation of the leg* (to diminish the edema)
  – *immobilization* (because of the danger of embolism)
- Later – *compression* (to improve the venous return)

**Specific treatment**

| Procedure | Indication | Contraindications |
|---|---|---|
| **Thrombectomy** | Phlegmasia cerulea dolens threatening gangrene danger of lung embolus When thrombolysis is contraindicated After unsuccessful thrombolysis In fresh thrombosis (max. 4–5 days old) In fresh thrombosis with floating thrombus (against embolism danger) | Old thrombi with vein wall adhesion (Endothelial damage – high recurrence rate) High general operative risk in poor general condition Infection of the operative field Elderly Malignancy Previous post-thrombotic syndrome Only a slight probability of the development of a post-thrombotic syndrome (e.g. isolated leg thrombosis) |
| **Thrombolysis** (very high short-term lysis) | Acute thrombosis up to 1 week old (older thrombosis up to 3 weeks old) | Acute gastric or colorectal ulcer Recent major operation History of CNS trauma or insult Hemorrhagic diathesis Hypertension Endocarditis Elderly Malignancy Pregnancy |
| **Anti-coagulation** | After lysis or thrombectomy When lysis and thrombectomy contraindicated In older thrombosis to avoid thrombus growth In isolated leg vein thrombosis | |

# VASCULAR SURGERY AND THE LYMPHATIC SYSTEM

## Varicose veins: diagnosis and treatment

**Trendelenburg test**
- For determination of valve function of the major veins
- For proof of insufficiency of the perforating veins

**Patient standing**
Identify and mark the junction of
the great saphenous and femoral veins

**Patient lying down**
a) Leg lifted until vein empty. Stretch the empty vein. Compress venous junction tubing with a tourniquet

**Patient standing**
b) Observe the varices during 10–15 s of junction compression
c) Then release the compression

**During compression** (b)
Absent or only slow filling from the distal end: valves of the saphenous and communicating veins are **working** (bI)
Rapid filling from proximal to distal: valves of the saphenous or communicating veins **insufficient** (bII)

**After loosening the compression**
No additional filling from the groin. Junction valve of the great saphenous vein functional:
**Trendelenburg-negative**

Rapid additional filling from the groin: junction valve of the greater saphenous vein inadequate:
**Trendelenburg-positive** (c)

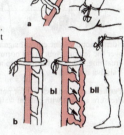
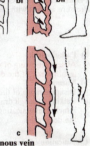

**Hach's classification of the trunk varicosities of the great saphenous vein**
I  Insufficiency limited to the groin area
II Distal insufficiency point a handbreadth proximal to the knee joint
III Distal insufficiency point a handbreadth distal from the knee joint
IV Insufficiency extending to the foot

**Frequent location of perforating veins**

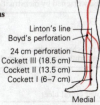
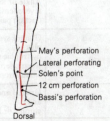

Medial:
- Dodd group
- Linton's line
- Boyd's perforation
- 24 cm perforation
- Cockett III (18.5 cm)
- Cockett II (13.5 cm)
- Cockett I (6–7 cm)

Dorsal:
- May's perforation
- Lateral perforating
- Solen's point
- 12 cm perforation
- Bassi's perforation

# MEMORIX SURGERY

**Doppler sonographic examination**
(From Schwilden, E.D. (1990))

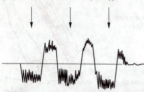

Normal sonographic current signal over the femoral vein in (a) normal breathing, (b) forced respiration and (c) Valsalva manuver

Retrograde flow in the great saphenous vein in the Valsalva manuver (↓) in consequence of insufficiency of the junction valve

**Perthes' test:** (indirect test for patency of the deep veins)
Pressure applied with patient walking about

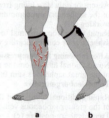

a) **Pathological:**
Absent emptying of varices in insufficiency of the deep veins
b) **Normal:**
Disappearance of the varices on walking, through drainage via the intact communicating veins and the deep veins

**Classification of chronic venous insufficiency in the lower extremity**
(After Widmar, Basle)

| Chronic venous insufficiency, Stage | Symptoms (uni- or bilateral) |
|---|---|
| I | Ankle or leg edema; severe tension-pain in the legs; traction pain (may be worsened by menstruation or pregnancy) |
| II | Grade I symptoms plus dystrophic skin changes; siderosclerosis, yellow-ochre purpura; white atrophy, pachyderma, acro-angiodermatitis, hypodermia |
| III | Grade I and II and chronic or healed-over crural ulcer |

# VASCULAR SURGERY AND THE LYMPHATIC SYSTEM

**Treatment of varicose veins**
**Access routes**
- Skin incision in the inguinal flexure
- Skin incision 2–3 cm above the inguinal groove (cosmetic advantages, preservation of the lymph vessels)

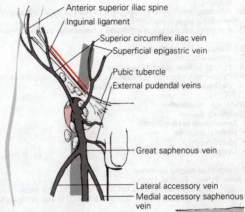

**Before ligature of the great saphenous vein ensure that the femoral vein is not stenosed**

**Treatment of inadequate perforating veins**
- Excision of the perforating veins
- Subfascial ligature of perforating veins

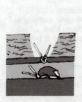
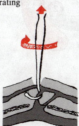

**Babcock's vein-stripping technique:**
After central ligature the great saphenous vein is extracted using an intraluminal vein stripper.

# Hodgkin's and non-Hodgkin's lymphoma

## Ann Arbor classification
I   Affecting a single lymph node group or a single extralymphatic organ
II  Affecting two or more lymph node groups on the same side of the diaphragm or one or more node groups and an extralymphatic organ on the same side of the diaphragm.
III Affecting lymph node groups on both sides of the diaphragm, possibly extralymphatic organs, possibly the spleen involved
IV  Extralymphatic organ involvement – bone, bone marrow, hepatic, etc.

E   Extranodal involvement
S   Spleen affected
A   Patient without general symptoms
B   Patient with generalized symptoms: fever >38°C, weight loss of more than 10% of the body weight in the previous 6 months

## Histologic classification of Hodgkin's disease
- Lymphocyte predominance
- Nodular sclerosis
- Mixed type
- Lymphocyte depletion

## Procedure in staging operation
(From Siewert, R. *et al.* (1979))
Staging surgical procedures are not often indicated with present imaging technology, and then only in specific cases. It is not indicated in non-Hodgkin's lymphoma)

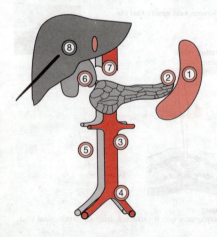

① Splenectomy
② Lymph node excision at the splenic hilus
③ Left para-aortic lymph node excision
④ Left iliac lymph node excision
⑤ Mesenteric root node excision
⑥ Hepatoduodenal ligament area lymph node excision
⑦ Celiac trunk lymph node excision
⑧ Liver biopsy

# VASCULAR SURGERY AND THE LYMPHATIC SYSTEM

## Classification of lymphoid neoplasms
(Adapted from *Blood*, Vol. 84, No. 5, September 1, 1994: pp 1361–1392)

**Non-Hodgkin's lymphomas**
### B-cell neoplasms
I. **Precursor B-cell neoplasms:** precursor B-lymphoblastic leukemia/lymphoma (low-grade)
II. **Peripheral B-cell neoplasms**
  - B-cell chronic lymphocytic leukemia/non-Hodgkin's lymphoma, small lymphocytic type (low-grade)
  - Lymphoplasmacytoid lymphoma (e.g. Waldenstroms macroglobulinemia)
  - Mantle cell lymphoma
  - Follicular center cell lymphoma
    Follicular small cleaved cell type (low-grade)
    Follicular mixed cell type (low-grade)
    Follicular large cell type (intermediate-grade)
  - Marginal zone B-cell lymphoma
    Low-grade B-cell lymphoma of mucosal associated lymphoid tissue or 'MALT'-type (low-grade)
    'monocytoid B-cell' lymphoma (low-grade)
  - Hairy cell leukemia
  - Large cell B-cell lymphoma, diffuse (both intermediate and high-grade subtypes)
  - Burkitt's lymphoma (high-grade) and high-grade B-cell lymphoma, Burkitt's-like
  - Plasmacytoma/multiple myeloma

### T-cell neoplasms
I. **Precursor T-cell neoplasms:** precursor T-cell lymphoblastic lymphoma / leukemia
II. **Peripheral T-cell and NK cell neoplasms**
  - T-cell chronic lymphocytic leukemia/prolymphocytic leukemia (rare)
  - Large granular lymphocyte leukemia (LGL)
  - Mycosis fungoides/Sezary syndrome
  - Peripheral T-cell lymphomas (including lymphoepithelioid cell Lennert's-type lymphoma)
  - Angioimmunoblastic T-cell lymphoma (AILD-like)
  - Angiocentric T-cell lymphoma
  - Intestinal T-cell lymphoma
  - Adult T-cell leukemia/lymphoma
  - Anaplastic large cell lymphoma (CD 30 or 'Ki-1' positive anaplastic lymphoma)
  - Other

**Hodgkin's disease:**
Lymphocyte predominance
Nodular sclerosis
Mixed cellularity
Lymphocyte depleted

| Grade | Histopathological/pathological type |
|---|---|
| Low grade | Small lymphocytic (SL)<br>Follicular, predominantly small cleared cell (FSC)<br>Follicular, mixed small cleared, large-cell (FM) |
| Intermediate grade | Follicular, predominantly large<br>Diffuse, small cleared cell<br>Diffuse, mixed small and large cell<br>Diffuse, large cell: cleared or non-cleared cell |
| High grade | Immunoblastic<br>Lymphoblastic: convoluted or non-convoluted cell<br>Small non-cleared cell: Burkitt's or non-Burkitt's |
| Miscellaneous | Mycosis fungoides<br>Sezary syndrome<br>Multiple myeloma/solitary plasmacytoma |

In non-Hodgkin's lymphoma, the histologic type and classification is of more prognostic significance than the stage.

# MEMORIX SURGERY

## The unconscious patient

**Management of the unconscious patient – immediate measures**
- Adequate oxygenation – clearance of the respiratory passages?, spontaneous breathing?, intubation required?
- Check pulse and blood pressure, resuscitation SOS
- Insert intravenous drip, take blood for laboratory examination, drug screening
- Glucose administration (later thiamin and/or naloxone)
- Fluid replacement, further review of the cardiopulmonary state and laboratory tests
- Insert bladder catheter, check excretion
- High cerebral pressure (hyperventilation, mannitol, steroids)
- Seizures (diazepam, lorazepam) (I.V.)
- If meningitis suspected, lumbar puncture (Gram stain, bacteriological examination)
- Positioning (see page 47)

**Etiology**
– Accident
– Internal or neurological causes

**Pathophysiological causes**
**Supratentorial area**
often associated hemiplegia, focal neurological signs, conjugated eye deviation from the hemiplegic side with small reactive pupils, Cheyne–Stokes breathing
**Infratentorial area**
focal neurological signs, hemiplegia, conjugated eye deviation of the hemiplegic side possible, abnormal pupil reaction
**Metabolic disorders**
symmetrical motor disorders, small normally reacting pupils, conjugated eye deviation (exceptions: drugs, self-administered opiates with tiny reactive pupils, wide fixed pupils from atropine, active pupils from glutathimidine)
**Psychic disorders**
inconspicuous neurological findings associated with breathing, pupillary reaction, pattern of reflexes, normal rapid physiological nystagmus to the opposite side on stimulation of the tympanic membrane with 10 ml of ice water, normal EEG

**Clinical examination**
- Vital functions (mechanical, Cheyne–Stokes, gasping respiration, apnea)
- Heart/circulation (shock, resuscitation)
- Consciousness (sleepiness, stupor, coma)
- Reaction on questioning
- Spontaneous motor reaction on the affected side
- Pupillary reaction
- Skin color

# NEUROSURGERY

## Glasgow coma and outcome scales

### Glasgow coma scale
(From Teasdale and Jennett (1976))

|  |  | Points |
|---|---|---|
| **Eye opening** | Spontaneous | 4 |
|  | On questioning | 3 |
|  | On painful irritation | 2 |
|  | None | 1 |
| **Verbal reaction** | Orientated | 5 |
|  | Confused | 4 |
|  | Single words | 3 |
|  | Sounds | 2 |
|  | None | 1 |
| **Motor reaction** | After requests | 6 |
|  | Targeted pain reaction | 5 |
|  | Flexor mechanism | 4 |
|  | Atypical flexor reaction | 3 |
|  | Extensor mechanism | 2 |
|  | None | 1 |
| Maximum points |  | 15 |
| Minimum points |  | 3 |

### Glasgow outcome scale
(After Jennett and Bond (1975))

1. Death: (without return of consciousness after the brain lesion)
2. Apallic syndrome: (coma vigile, 'vegetative state') – non-reactive to speech, open eyes, vegetative function intact)
3. Severe disablement: patient is dependent on a third person because of his or her physical and/or mental handicaps
4. Moderate disablement: patient is independent with daily help, can travel by public transport and can work in a protecting workshop, but is clearly handicapped
5. Minimal handicap: return to normal life with only slight neurological defect after normal recovery

**Note:**
Always note the time and date of the examination (days after the brain damage).
If possible, make a daily record of the physical and mental condition.

The Glasgow outcome scale was developed for the assessment of the condition of the individual categories of skull–brain trauma. A further application of value is its application to the assessment of patient state after secondary brain damage, encephalitis or spontaneous cerebral hemorrhage.

# MEMORIX SURGERY

## Disorders of consciousness
**Differential diagnosis of intra- and extracranial causes**
(After Berlit (1992))

|  | Slowly increasing consciousness disorder | Sudden loss of consciousness | Increasing confusion |
|---|---|---|---|
| **Intracranial origin** | | | |
| Trauma | Subdural hematoma | Epidural hematoma Contusion | Post-traumatic psychosis Subdural hematoma |
| Tumor | Edema | Interior compression, internal bleeding, occlusive hydrocephalus | Edema |
| Vascular | Space-occupying Infarct Intracerebral bleeding | Brainstem infarct, hypertension, massive bleeding, sub-arachnoid hemorrhage | Edema after infarct Bleeding Transitory global amnesia |
| Inflammation | Bacterial meningitis Encephalitis | Pressure from brain abscess, internal bleeding or edema from encephalitis | Encephalitis |
| Toxic | Central pontine myelinolysis Wernicke encephalopathy | Central pontine myelinolysis, corpus callosum degeneration | Wernicke encephalopathy Alcohol delirium Korsakow syndrome Alcoholic hallucinations |
| Epilepsy | | Grand mal frontal-lobe faint | Twilight state Psychomotor attacks |
| **Extracranial origin** | | | |
| Metabolic | Electrolyte disorders (Na, K) Acidosis/alkalosis Uremia, liver failure | Electrolyte disorder (Ca, Na) Porphyria | Electrolyte imbalance Anorexia Hyper/hypothermia Porphyria |
| Hormonal | Hyperglycemia Hyperthyroidism Hypopituitarism | Hyperglycemia Hypoglycemia | Hyperglycemia Hypoglycemia Hyperthyroidism |
| Heart / circulation | Blood loss, anemia | Low blood pressure Cardiac rhythm disorder Carotid sinus syndrome | Anemia |
| Lungs | Hypoventilation | Pulmonary embolus | |
| Psychiatric | Catatonia | Psychogenic faints | Dementia |
| Toxic | Sedatives, hypnotics Thymoleptics Neuroleptics Anti-convulsives CO | Sedatives, hypnotics Drugs | Drugs |

# NEUROSURGERY

## Craniocerebral trauma

- Careful history/reconstruction of the circumstances
- Clinical examination, inspection and revision of the wound
- X-rays of skull in several planes, possibly CT
- If dura is injured (loss of liquor, destroyed cerebral tissue) – operation indicated
- Complications after incomplete operative repair: meningitis, cerebral abscess, psychic changes
- In depressed fracture of more than a skull's thickness – operation indicated

### Classification of craniocerebral trauma

|  | I (light) | II (medium severity) | III (severe) |
|---|---|---|---|
| Unconsciousness | ≤15 min | ≤1 h | >1 h |
| Disorders of consciousness | ≤1 h | ≤24 h | >24 h |
| Accompanying symptoms | Headache, nausea, vertigo, retrograde, amnesia | Fleeting pareses or pyramidal tract signs, meningismus (subarachnoid hemorrhage) | Pareses, pyramidal tract signs, motor unrest, cerebral coma, disorders of vital function |
| EEG changes | Short-term, slight general changes possible | Marked general changes | Severe general and focal changes |
| Progress | Distinct improvement after a few days | Better after days–3 weeks CAUTION: brain edema, intracerebral bleeding | Usually cerebral edema, convulsions CAUTION: midbrain syndrome |
| Prognosis | Complete recovery | Mostly complete cure, possibly remaining disorders | Almost always residual symptoms, as post-traumatic epilepsy |
| Treatment | Short-term bed rest | Prophylaxis against brain edema and/or intracerebral bleeding | Intensive therapy, prevention of complications, operative intervention SOS |

# Clinical staging of craniocerebral trauma

|  |  | Midbrain syndrome | | | | Bulbar-brain syndrome | |
|---|---|---|---|---|---|---|---|
|  |  | I | II | III | IV | I | II |
| Conscious |  | Sleepiness | Coma | Coma | Coma | Coma | Coma |
| Reaction to | Accoustic irritation | Turns to target | None Untargeted | None Extended limbs | None Extension automatism | None Stretch automatism | None None |
| Oculomotor | Eye | Normal | Swimming movements | Divergent | Divergent | Fixed Divergent | Fixed Divergence |
|  | Pupils | Mid-open | Mid-open | Below mid-open | Below mid-open ↓↓ | Wide | Wide |
|  | Reaction to light | Prompt | ↓ | ↓ | ↓↓ | None | None |
| Brainstem reflexes | Oculocephalic reflex | Slight | Puppet-head+ | Puppet-head+ | Slight | None | None |
|  | Cliospinal reflex | + | + | + | (+) | None | None |
|  | Vestibulo-ocular reflex | + | + | Tonic reaction to cold irritation | Only ipsilateral | None | None |
| Body movements | Posture | Normal | Legs outstretched Legs raised | Bend-stretch posture | Extended posture ↑↑ | Extended legs ↑ | Sleeping |
|  | Tone | Normal | Bulk movements of arm | Bend-stretch synergism | Stretch-synergism + | Stretch-synergism + | Sleeping |
|  | Spontaneous movements | Bulk movements | (+) |  |  |  | – |
|  | Babinski | – |  | + |  |  | – |
| Vegetative system | Respiration | Irregular | Possibly Cheyne-Stokes | ↑ | Mechanical respiration | | None |
|  | Pulse | (↑) | (↑) | ↑↑↑ | ↑↑ | ↑↑ | →←→ |
|  | Blood pressure | Normal | (↑) | ↑↑ | ↑↑ | ↑↑ |  |
|  | Temperature | Normal | (↑) |  | ↑↑ | ↑↑ | Normal ↓ |

# NEUROSURGERY

(After Lücking, C.H. (1976))

| Phases of brain-stem damage | Midbrain syndrome | | | | Bulbar syndrome | |
|---|---|---|---|---|---|---|
| | 1 | 2 | 3 | 4 | 1 | 2 |
| Vigilance | Sleepiness | Stupor | Coma | Coma | Coma | Coma |
| Reactivity | Retarded | Reduced | Absent | Absent | Absent | Absent |
| Spontaneous motor activity | | | | | | |
| Motor pain reaction | | | | | | |
| Muscle tone | Normal | Arm support | Raised | Raised ++ | Normal-lax | Lax |
| Pupil width | | | | | | |
| Pupil reaction to light | | | | | | |
| Eye movement | Oscillating | Dysjointed | Absent | Absent | Absent | Absent |
| Oculocerebral reflex | ∅ | + | ++ | + | | |
| Vestibular reflex | Normal +++ | +++ | Tonic | Dissociated | ∅ | ∅ |
| Breathing | | | | | | |
| Temperature | Normal | Normal | Slightly + | Definitely raised | Reduced | Reduced ↑↑ |
| Pulse rate | | | | | | |
| Blood pressure | | | | | | |

**Estimation scale for pupil width assessment (mm)**

2  3  4  5  6  7  8  9

# MEMORIX SURGERY

## Cerebral arteries and collaterals

**Important collaterals of the vessels supplying the brain**

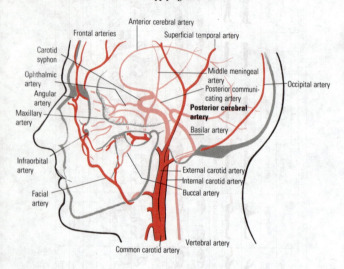

**Internal–external circulation:**
Ophthalmic artery

**Anterior (carotid)–posterior (vertebrobasilar) circulation:**

Posterior communicating artery (Posterior siphon)
Choroidal artery (posterior siphon)
Occipital artery (external vertebral)
Leptomeningeal anastomoses (anteroposterior, middle posterior)

**Right–left hemisphere:**

Anterior communicating artery (anterior right–anterior left)

# Aneurysms

## Common sites of cerebral aneurysms

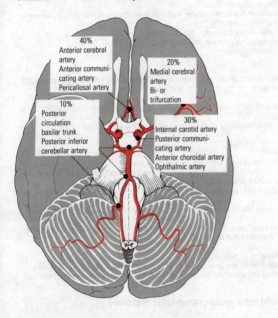

- 40% Anterior cerebral artery / Anterior communicating artery / Pericallosal artery
- 20% Medial cerebral artery / Bi- or trifurcation
- 10% Posterior circulation basilar trunk / Posterior inferior cerebellar artery
- 30% Internal carotid artery / Posterior communicating artery / Anterior choroidal artery / Ophthalmic artery

**Pathogenesis**
Paralytic (through cerebral nerve compression) – rare
Rupture

**Treatment**
Metal clip
'Trapping' procedures
Intravascular occlusion

# MEMORIX SURGERY

## Classification of subarachnoid hemorrhage
(After Hunt, W.E. and Hess, R.M. (1968))

I   Mild headache, mild meningism
II  Moderate to severe headache, severe meningismus, cranial nerve paresis, no wider neurological involvement
III Drowsiness, mild focal deficiency, psychic changes
IV  Stupor, hemiparesis, vegetative dysregulation
V   Coma, midbrain symptoms

### Diagnosis
- Clinical picture: disorders of consciousness, sudden onset of headache, neck rigidity, vertigo, vomiting
- CT
- Spinal puncture: blood-stained fluid (Caution: danger of compression – aspiration of a few ml only)
- Angiography: demonstration of the source of bleeding and of other vascular anomalies

### Course:
*Recurrent bleeding* frequent, prognosis increasingly worse
*Vascular spasm* as a local protective mechanism can cause ischemia in dependent parts → brain edema, rise of intracranial pressure
*Mass displacement* and brainstem compression can follow brain edema or intracerebral bleeding
*Ventricle tamponade:* bleeding into the ventricle → coma, fixed pupils, rigidity (poor prognosis)
*Bleeding into the basal cisterns* → spasm of the basal central rami → ischemia of the vital autonomic center of the hypothalamus

### Time for operation
As soon as possible after resolution of the acute symptoms, to prevent recurrence
In space-occupying intracerebral hemorrhage immediate operation may be indicated

## The basal cisterns – diagrammatic (lateral)

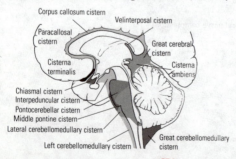

# NEUROSURGERY

## Intracerebral space-occupying lesions

### Hemorrhage
Extradural (between the internal table of the skull and the dura mater), often after injury to the middle meningeal artery – transverse temporal fracture, homolateral pupil widening, contralateral pyramidal tract symptomatology

Acute subdural (between dura mater and soft meninges), after destruction of brain tissue and tearing of arachnoidal and cortical vessels, often following severe brain damage, mostly difficult to diagnose because of the accompanying injuries

Chronic subdural, unspecific symptoms, differential diagnosis: tumor, cerebrovascular insult

Subarachnoid, after rupture of subarachnoid vessels, neck rigidity

### Hygroma
Post-traumatic subdural fluid collection

### Cerebral abscess

### Tumors of the nervous system and their sites
(From Berlit (1991))

| Brain | | Spinal cord |
|---|---|---|
| Supratentorial | Infratentorial | |
| Hemispheres:<br>Multiform glioblastoma<br>Astrocytoma<br>Aligodendroglioma<br>Meningioma<br>Metastases | Adults:<br>Acoustic neuroma<br>Metastases<br>Meningioma<br>Angioblastoma (Lindau) | Extradural:<br>Metastases<br>Dermoid<br><br>Intradural extramedullary:<br>Meningioma<br>Neurinoma<br>Angioma |
| Midline:<br>Pituitary tumors<br>Pineal tumors<br>Craniopharyngiomas | Children:<br>Cerebellar astrocytoma<br>Medullary blastoma<br>Ependymoma<br>Brainstem glioma | Intradural intramedullary:<br>Ependymoma<br>Astrocytoma<br>Metastases |

### Signs of brain pressure
- Feeling of pressure in the head
- Headache
- Nausea, vomiting
- Disc congestion on ophthalmoscopy
- Psychic disturbances
- Blurring of consciousness and awareness
- Cranial nerve disorders (e.g. abducens nerve, double vision, oculomotor nerve, dilated pupils)
- Vital function disorders (Cheyne–Stokes respiration, mechanical respiration, gasping)

# MEMORIX SURGERY

## Hydrocephalus

**Definition:** Pathological enlargement of the cerebral ventricles

**Causes:**
- Blockage of the drainage canals (see figure) by malformation, stenosis, tumor, etc. (occlusive hydrocephalus)
- Damage to the absorption surfaces, disproportion between fluid production and resorption from meningitis, subarachnoid bleeding, birth trauma, result of injury (hydrocephalus communicans)

**Clinical picture:** Pathologically enlarged head increase, growth and bulging of the fontanelles, gaping of the sutures, the 'twilight phenomenon' (pupils partially covered by the lower lid), venous congestion of the head, brain pressure symptoms

**Treatment:**
- Removal of the cause (e.g. tumor)
- Temporary or permanent CSF diversion (ventriculoatrial shunt, ventriculoperitoneal shunt)

### Common causes of drainage disorder
(From Bettex, M., Kuffer, F. and Scharli, A.F. (1975))

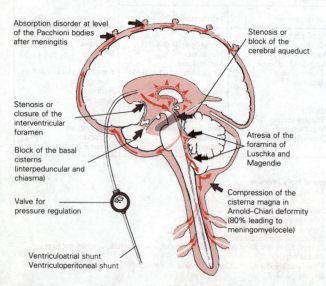

# NEUROSURGERY

## Segment innervation

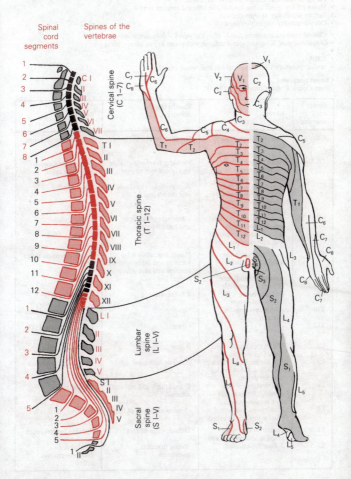

# MEMORIX SURGERY

## Spinal emergencies

- Partial or complete effects distal to the lesion
- Motor effects: quiet at the level of the affected anterior horn
- Surface sensibility: sharply defined
- Deep sensibility: vaguely defined

- Clinical examination immediately after the injury – documentation!
- Diagnostic aids: X-rays of spinal column with plates in two planes, erect
- CT
- NMR
- lumbar puncture – bleeding?, transit into spinal canal?

**Clinical symptoms**
(From Oppel, F. and Conzen, M. (1990))

| Spinal cord segment | Motor | Results (levels) Sensory | Reflex |
|---|---|---|---|
| C4 | Head lifting possible Quadriplegia Diaphragmatic breathing | Shoulder level and clavicle | Scapulohumeral reflex |
| C5, C6 | Intact trapezius, weak external rotation of arm otherwise quadriplegia | Shoulder level and clavicle and lateral side of arm | Biceps reflex, radial periosteal reflex |
| C7 | Arm abduction and flexion at elbow possible, elbow extension deficient | Arm midline, radial side and thumb free | Triceps reflex |
| C8 | Upper arm and shoulder muscles free, finger flexors, thumb extensors and interossei paralyzed | Ulnar side of forearm and hand free | Thumb reflex |
| T1 | Arms free up to the small hand muscles | Hands free, ulnar edge forearm and inner forearm and arm affected | Finger extension reflex |
| T4 | Arms and hands free, sitting up impossible | Nipple line | |
| T8 | Corresponding intercostal nerves | Rib curvature | Epigastric reflex |
| T10 | Abdominal muscles affected | Navel | Upper abdominal skin reflex |
| T12 | | Groin | Lower abdominal skin reflex |
| L2 | Hip flexors and femoral adductors paretic | Below groin | Cremaster reflex |
| L3 | Hip flexion free, little leg adduction, the other leg muscles paretic | Anterior and inner side of thigh free | Patellar tendon reflex |
| L4 | Knee extension little affected, femoral and foot muscles paretic | Dorsal thigh and leg–foot affected | Gluteal reflex |
| L5 | Quadriceps unaffected, plantar flexion disturbed | Outside and back of foot | Posterior tibial reflex |
| S1 | Plantar flexion not possible, micturition and defecation affected | Outside edge of foot | Achilles tendon reflex |
| S2–5 | | Riding breeches anesthesia | Anal reflex Bulbocavernosus reflex |

# NEUROSURGERY

## Spinal injuries and treatment

### Crutchfield extension (see figure)
- Immobilizing the cervical spinal column in extension (traction 1–15 kg) according to the fixation of the dislocation
- Take a lateral X-ray after each adjustment or increase in the traction
- Alternative to the Crutchfield extension: immobilization in a plastic collar or a Halovest

**Application:**
1 cm above the auricle at the level of the external auditory canal, avoiding perforation beyond the **superficial** skull table

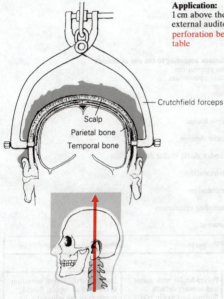

### Operative procedures
Dependent on the fracture, particularly in producing the anticipated stability
Ventral fusion with vertebral disc extraction. Spondylodesis with bone cement or autologous bone chips, plate fixation
Vertebral body substitution plasty in fragmented fractures. Replacement with autologous corticospongious chips. Plate splinting
Dorsal fixation with clamps, wire, chip bone, etc.
Screwing of the axis in axis fracture from the front, with additional screwing of C1,C2 from behind

# MEMORIX SURGERY

## Peripheral nerve lesions

### Sensory nerve damage
- Sweat gland hypersecretion (partial lesion)
- Deficiency in sweat secretion (complete lesion)
- Disorders of superficial sensibility (pain, temperature)
- Paresthesia (partial lesion)
- Anesthesia (complete lesion)

### Classification of motor nerve lesions
M0  No muscular activity
M1  Visible contractions, no function
M2  Movement possible after elimination of gravity
M3  Movement possible against moderate resistance
M4  Movement possible against gravity
M5  Normal strength

### Millesi classification of nerve lesions according to the site of fibrosis
A  Fibrosis of the epifascicular epineurium
B  Fibrosis of the interfascicular epineurium
C  Fibrosis of the endoneurium
N  Neuroma
X  Scar

### Sunderland classification of nerve lesions
1. Neurapraxia
   Conduction block from myelin damage
2. Axonotmesis I
   Interruption of the axis cylinder, distal Waller degeneration
3. Axonotmesis II
   Additional lesion of the endoneurium
4. Axonotmesis III
   Additional lesion of the perineurium
5. Neurotmesis
   Complete nerve division including epineurium

### Differential diagnosis and treatment

| Root lesion | Plexus lesion | Peripheral nerve lesion |
|---|---|---|
| **Diagnosis** | | |
| Root pain, mono or polyradicular; empty, ruptured or puffed root pockets, cyst formation in NMR or myelography | Polyradicular with motor and sensory defects Normal findings in NMR and myelography | Loss or partial loss of sensation in the area of supply, flaccid paralysis of the relevant muscles, muscle atrophy in prolonged cases |
| **Treatment** | | |
| No reconstruction muscle transfer operations possible | Reconstruction with cable interposition muscle transfer operations possible | Nerve suture, with cable interposition (e.g. from the sural nerve) Muscle transfer operations possible |

# NEUROSURGERY

## Peripheral nerve compression syndromes

### Examples:
- Carpal tunnel syndrome – median nerve compression underneath the transverse carpal ligament at the wrist
- Cubital tunnel syndrome – ulnar nerve compression over the medial epicondyle at the elbow
- Ulnar nerve entrapment in Guyon's canal – ulnar nerve compression at the wrist
- Radial tunnel syndrome – compression from radial head to the supinator muscle
- Posterior interosseous branch of the radial nerve – compression as it passes around the lateral elbow and enters the supinator muscle beneath the Arcade of Frohse

### Symptoms
- Pain at the site of compression which may radiate
- Numbness and tingling which may progress to loss of sensation
- Muscle atrophy due to axon death, often prolonged compression

### Diagnosis
- Clinical neurological examination
- Electrophysiological examination, e.g. electromyography (EMG), motor and sensory nerve conduction velocity (NCV), somatosensory evoked potential (SEP)
- Sweat test

### Radiological diagnosis
- X-rays
- Computed tomography (CT)
- MRI

### Treatment
- Conservative, e.g. splinting, mobilization, anti-inflammatory medication
- Operative, e.g. nerve decompression, external neurolysis

# MEMORIX SURGERY

## Disc prolapse

### Sites of lumbosacral disc hernias

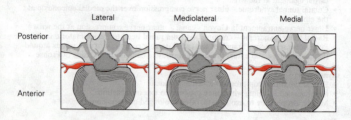

### Indications for operation

**Absolute:**
Acute motor paralysis, motor function loss on important muscle groups, incipient cauda syndrome

**No indication**
Long-standing muscular pareses without other complaints

**Relative:**
Failure of previous conservative treatment for the root syndrome with severe pain, insignifant functional muscular paresis, with anticipated inability to work for a prolonged period under conservative treatment

### Contraindications
Doubtful diagnosis, absent root symptoms, unwillingness on the part of the patient

### Common root compression syndrome resulting from intervertebral disc prolapse
(From Berlit, P. (1992))

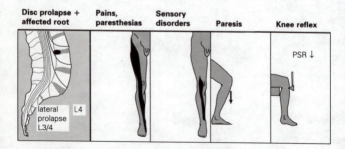

# NEUROSURGERY

**Common root compression syndrome resulting from intervertebral disc prolapse (From Berlit, P. (1992))**

| Disc prolapse + affected root | Pain, paresthesia | Sensation affected | Paresis | Leg reflex |
|---|---|---|---|---|
| Lateral prolapse L4/5 — L6 | | | Heel stand ↓ | Tibialis-posterior reflex ↓ |
| Lateral prolapse L5/Sp — S1 | | | Toe stand ↓ | ASR ↓ |
| Medial prolapse L4/5 **Cauda equina** | | | Bladder–rectum paralysis, breeches anesthesia, bilateral leg paralysis | ASR ↓ |

## Brain death criteria

**Assumptions**
- Primary brain damage (supra-, infratentorial
- Examples: most severe brain injury, intracranial hemorrhage, cerebral infarct, malignant tumor, acute obstructive hydrocephalus
- Secondary brain damage as a result of hypoxia, cardiovascular conditioned circular conditioned circulatory arrest, shock

**Exclude:**
- Intoxication (association with cerebral circulatory arrest is proven)
- Neuromuscular block
- Freezing
- Circulatory shock
- Endocrine coma
- Metabolic coma

**Symptoms/findings (two independent examiners, not associated with a transplantation team)**
- Unconsciousness
- Dilated pupils (slight, medium)
- Eliminate mydriatic drug cause
- No oculocephalic reflex obtainable
- No corneal reflex obtainable
- No reaction to painful stimulus in the trigeminal area (e.g. nasal septum)
- No pharyngeal reflex obtainable (e.g. by aspiration)
- No spontaneous respiration (negative apnea test, 60 mmHg obligatory)

**Supplementary investigations**
- EEG, isoelectric (0-line) over 30 min in adults
- Brainstem auditory evoked responses
- Median SEP: no reaction above neck line
- Doppler sonography
- Bilateral angiography
- Aortic arch DSA
- Demonstration of cerebral circulatory arrest
- Nuclear medicine: brain flow study

**Observation time**
- Adults with primary brain damage: 12 h
- Adults with secondary brain damage: 72 h
- Children with primary brain damage: 24 h
- Early newborn with primary brain damage: 72 h

**Time of death – time of establishment of final diagnosis**

**International Brain Death Criteria**
(Modified from Frowein *et al.* (1985))

|  | Germany, 1991 | USA, 1981 | GB, 1976 | Switzerland, 1983 |
|---|---|---|---|---|
| **Presumption** | | | | |
| Diagnosis | + | + | + | + |
| No intoxication | + | + | + | + |
| No hypothermia | + | + | + | + |
| No hypovolemia | + | + | + | + |
| **Clinically** | | | | |
| Coma | + | + | + | + |
| Apnea test | + | + | + | + |
| (pCO$_2$, mmHg) | >60 | >60 | >50 | >50 |
| Mydriasis dilatation | + | + | + | + |
| Brainstem reflex | + | + | + | + |
| Signatures | 2 | 1 | 2 | 1 |
| **Observation time (h)** | | | | |
| In primary brain damage | 12 | 12 | 6 | 6 |
| In secondary brain damage | 72 | 24 | 12 | 48 |
| **Additional** | | | | |
| EEG, no response | 30 min | 6 h/30 min | – | 2 in 24 h |
| AEP fall out | + | – | – | – |
| Circulatory arrest | Angiography | Nuclear medicine | – | Angiography |
| ICP above systolic RR | – | Brain flow study | – | + |

# ONCOLOGY

## Condition of the cancer patient

**Performance status**
**Karnofsky scale**

- 100% Normal, no complaints, no sign of illness
- 90% Capable of normal activities, slight signs or symptoms of illness
- 80% Normal activities with fatigue possible, few signs or symptoms of illness
- 70% Cares for him or herself, incapable of normal activities or normal work
- 60% Occasional support needed at work, can attend to most needs personally
- 50% Considerable support required, frequent medical attention necessary
- 40% Handicapped, requires special care and support
- 30% Severely disabled, hospital admission required, although there is as yet no danger of death
- 20% Very ill, hospital admission necessary, active medical support needed
- 10% Moribund
- 0 Death

**Zubrod scale**

- 0 Normal activity
- 1 Symptoms but ambulatory and able to carry out daily activities
- 2 Out of bed more than 50% of time, occasionally needs assistance
- 3 In bed more than 50% of time, needs skilled care
- 4 100% bedridden

Performance status should be evaluated each time the patient is seen during long-term follow-up

# MEMORIX SURGERY

## Cancer staging: TNM system
(From CUICC (1987))

| | | | |
|---|---|---|---|
| c | clinical (cT, cN, cM) | M1 OSS | Bones |
| p | pathological (pT, pN, pM) | M1 SKI | Skin |
| T | Tumor | M1 THO | Thorax |
| T0 | No support for tumor | | |
| Tis | Carcinoma *in situ* | M1 ... | Wider localization |
| T1–4 | Size of tumor | C | Diagnostic certainty |
| T(m) | Multiple organs involved T1(m) | C1 | Physical examination, X-rays |
| (T ...) | Multiple count in one organ T2(3) | C2 | CT, NMR, angiogram, lymphogram |
| TX | Size of tumor not certain | C3 | Cytology |
| TX a–d | Special subgroups | C4 | Surgical exploration and histologic examination (pTNM) |
| N | Lymph nodes affected | | |
| N0 | No lymph nodes affected | C5 | Autopsy |
| N1–3 | Extent of lymph node involvement | G | Histopathological grading |
| | | G1 | Well-differentiated |
| NX | Lymph node involvement not measureable | G2 | Moderately differentiated |
| | | G3 | Undifferentiated |
| M | Distant metastases | R0 | No residual tumor |
| M0 | No distant metastases | R1 | Microscopic tumor residual |
| M1 | Distant metastases | R2 | Macroscopic tumor residual |
| M1 ABD | Abdomen | r | Local recurrence (rpT 1) |
| M1 BRA | Brain | y | Intra/post-therapeutic stage classification (ypT) |
| M1 HEA | Head/neck | | |
| M1 HEP | Liver | | |

## Tumor therapy

### Morphological examination of microscopic sections

Cytology (assessment of cells): shape, size, nuclear size, nucleus–plasma relation, chromatin content of nuclei, establish integrity of examined cells

Histology (assessment of tissues): differentiation, proliferation, destruction of adjacent tissue, infiltration into neighboring tissues, invasion of blood and/or lymphatic vessels, mitosis count

**Establish integrity and extent of the investigated tissue, make diagnosis, make prognosis, e.g. TNM formula**

### Abbreviated Bethesda system of cervical PAP smear reporting

### Adequacy of the specimen
Satisfactory for evaluation
Satisfactory for evaluation by limited by ... (reason)
Unsatisfactory for evaluation ... (reason)

# ONCOLOGY

**General categorization** (optional)
  Within normal limits
  Descriptive diagnosis (which see)
**Descriptive diagnoses**
  Benign changes:
    Infections (specify)
    Reactive changes (describe abnormality likely to have caused changes)
  Epithelial cell abnormalities (squamous cell)
    Atypical squamous cells of undetermined significance (qualify)
    Low-grade squamous intraepithelial lesion (includes human papilloma virus
    infection and mild dysplasia)
    High-grade squamous intraepithelial lesion (includes moderate and severe
    dysplasia and carcinoma *in situ*, CIN II and III)
    Squamous cell carcinoma
  Epithelial cell abnormalities (glandular cells)
    Endometrial cells, benign, in a post-menopausal woman
    Atypical glandular cells of undetermined significance (qualify)
    Adenocarcinoma (endocervical, endometrial, other)
  Malignant neoplasm (NOS)
  Hormonal evaluation (lateral wall vaginal specimen only)

**Note:** clinical judgement is exercised in the follow-up of abnormalities. Any report of a squamous lesion of 'low grade' or greater should be followed by tissue examination. To repeat the PAP smear is not acceptable as an adequate form of follow-up once low-grade or higher squamous lesions have been reported. Atypical glandular cells of endocervical origin may be representative of adenocarcinoma *in situ* and must be followed with repeat PAP smear or tissue examination. Infections should be confirmed by specific microbiological testing.

**Contemporary tumor therapy generally follows the recommendations of the specialist working parties (AIO, CAO, etc.) or the conclusions of consensus conferences.**

**Preoperative:** radiotherapy, chemotherapy (for the improvement of operability and prognosis)

**Operative:**
- Curative ($R_0$)
- Attempted cure ($R_0$, $R_1$)
- Obtaining cells or tissue for diagnostic confirmation
- Evaluation of local and/or systemic (e.g. mediastinoscopy) extension
- Palliative ($R_1$, $R_2$)
    in an attempt at cure
    for improvement of quality of life
    to treat previous complications (e.g. intestinal obstruction, pathological fracture)
    removal of tumor-mediated complications
- Metastasis surgery

**Follow-up treatment**
- Supervision for freedom of local recurrence after curative operation
- Multimodal treatment after palliative operation or after operation with an unfavorable outlook (e.g. $T_3N_2G_2$)
- Constant critical consideration of the possible benefit of further measures in improvement of the patient's quality of life

# MEMORIX SURGERY

## Tumor markers

The different sensitivities and specificities for screening examination for the appropriate conditions

**Indication:** progress control, check on therapeutic success

**Clinically significant tumor markers**

|  | Normal value | Indications | Particulars |
|---|---|---|---|
| AFP (alpha fetoprotein) | <40 ng/ml | Hepatocellular carcinoma, germ cell tumor (non-seminoma) | Increased in neural tube defects, cirrhosis, chronic hepatitis |
| $B_2m$ ($B_2$-micro-globulin) | <2.0 mg/l | Multiple myeloma, NHL | Raised in renal diseases and AIDS |
| CA 15-3 | <28 U/ml | Breast cancer, ovarian carcinoma | Raised in liver cirrhosis |
| CA 19-9 | <7 U/l | Carcinoma of pancreas, colorectal carcinoma, gallbladder, bile duct carcinoma | Raised in cholelithiasis, pancreatitis, liver cirrhosis |
| CA 72-4 | <3 U/ml | Gastric carcinoma |  |
| CA 125 | <35 U/l | Ovarian, liver, pancreatic, lung carcinoma |  |
| Calcitonin (basal) | <19 pg/ml (male)<br><14 pg/ml (female) | Medullary thyroid carcinoma | >100 pg/ml warrants follow-up |
| CEA | <10 ng/ml | Colorectal carcinoma, stomach, breast, bronchial carcinoma |  |
| HCG | <5 IU/ml (female)<br><2.5 IU/ml (male) | Choriocarcinoma, seminoma (male 10%), hydatidiform mole | If both AFP and HCG initially positive, always repeat both |
| NSE (Neuron-specific enolase) | <12.5 ng/ml | Small-cell bronchial carcinoma, apudoma, neuroblastoma, Wilm's tumor | Centrifuge within 1 h |
| PSA (prostate-specific acid phosphatase) | 3.7 ng/ml<br>>40 to ≤4.0 ng/ml<br><40 to ≤2.7 ng/ml | Prostatic carcinoma | Blood test before rectal examination, tissue-specific, not tumor-specific |
| PAP (prostate-specific acid phosphatase) | <4 µg/ml | Prostatic carcinoma | Blood test before rectal examination, tissue-specific, not tumor-specific |
| SOC (squamous cell carcinoma antigen) | <2.5 ng/ml | Squamous cell carcinoma (lung, esophagus, HNO, uterus) | Raised by skin or salivary contamination |

# ONCOLOGY

## Tumor of unknown origin

**Definition:** cytologically or histologically confirmed malignancy, frequently as a metastatic lesion, primary site identified by normal investigational procedures

Frequency: 5–10% of all tumor disease,
Prognosis: often poor,
Diagnosis: primary tumor identified eventually in 15–27% of surviving patients
15% of cases remain without identification of the primary tumor until death

**Management:** therapy must be individualized to be successful

**The most common primary tumors with different metastatic location** (except hematologic or lymphatic neoplasms)
(From Jungi and Osterwalder (1990))

| Metastasis | Primary tumor |
| --- | --- |
| Lymph nodes | |
|   cervical | ENT, lung, thyroid |
|   supraclavicular | Breast, lung, gastrointestinal tract |
|   axillary | Breast, gastrointestinal tract |
|   inguinal | Urogenital, rectum |
|   retroperitoneal | Urogenital (including germ cell tumor) |
| | |
| Lung | Breast, kidney, thyroid |
| Bone | Breast, prostate, lung, kidney, thyroid |
| Bladder | Lung, breast |
| Skin | Skin, breast, lung |
| Liver | Gastrointestinal tract, pancreas, lung |
| Pleura | Lung, breast, ovary |
| Ascites | Gastrointestinal tract, ovary |

# MEMORIX SURGERY

## General – acute pain

**Diagnosis**
History
Examination
Additional findings
Further potential diagnostics

➤ **Diagnosis**

➤ **Treatment**

**Basic rules for pain therapy**
(From Zenz, M. (1984))

|  | Acute pain | Chronic pain |
|---|---|---|
| Aim | Freedom from pain | Freedom from pain |
| Duration | Short | Long |
| Application | Intravenous | Oral |
| Dosage | Determine individually | Determined individually |
| Intervals | As required | Regularly, prophylactically |
| Additional treatment | Seldom necessary | Regularly |

### Treatment of acute pain

**Warning and leading symptoms in acute illness:**
Treatment as required
Must not interfere with diagnosis

**Postoperative**

Wide variety in analgesic requirements between patients after similar operative procedures

Short-term repeat doses often necessary

**Medication:**

1. Non-opioid

2. Opioid (e.g. patient-controlled analgesia (PCA))
   Local anesthetic

3. Continuous regional anesthesia
   Epidural, catheter plexus anesthesia, e.g. in phantom pain prophylaxis

**Caution:** Opioid overdosage
Respiratory depression
Drowsiness

**Simple checking**

Respiration rate

Pulsoximetry

# TREATMENT OF PAIN

## Analgesics
### Non-opioid

| Drug | Administration | Single dose (mg) | Duration effect (h) | Single doses (per day) |
|---|---|---|---|---|
| Acetylsalicylic acid | i.v., p.o. | 1000 | 4–6 | 3–4 |
| Paracetamol | p.o., suppository | 1000 | 4–6 | 3–4 |
| Iboprufen | p.o., suppository | 400 | 4–6 | 3 |
| Ibuprofen retard | p.o. | 400 | 8–12 | 2 |
| Diclofenac | i.m., p.o., suppository | 50 | 2–6 | 3–4 |

### Opioid agonists, partial agonists and antagonists

| Drug | Equivalent (mg) | Administration | Single dose (mg) | Duration (h) | Dose interval in hours |
|---|---|---|---|---|---|
| **Mildly effective opioids** | | | | | |
| Codeine | 0.1–0.05 | p.o. | 30 | 4 | q 4 h |
| Dihydrocodeine retard | 0.1–0.05 | p.o. | 60 | 8–12 | q 8 h |
| Dextropropoxyphene | 0.1 | p.o. | 150 | 8–12 | q 4 h |
| Naloxone | | i.m., i.v. | 0.4 | 2–3 | q 2 h |
| **Strongly effective opioids** | | | | | |
| Morphine | 1 | p.o.-i.c.v. | 5–10 | 4 | 6 |
| Morphine sulphate (MST) | 1 | p.o. | 30 | 8–12 | 2–3 |
| MSR | 1 | Suppository | 30 | 6 | 6 |
| Laevomethadone | 3 | p.o., i.v., i.m. | 10 | 8–24 | 1 |
| Pethadine | 0.1 | i.v., i.m. | 50 | 2 | 12 |
| **Partial agonists** | | | | | |
| Pentazocine | 0.2 | i.v., i.m., p.o. | 30 | 3 | 8 |
| Buprenorphine | 40 | i.v., i.m., sl. | 0.2 | 6–8 | 3–4 |
| **Antagonists** | | | | | |
| Naloxone | 0 | i.v., i.m. | 2–4 | 2 | |
| Nalbuphine | 0.7 | i.v., i.m. | 4 | 4 | |

**Note:** Do not use combinations of opioid agonists and partial agonists because of the inability to assess the combined actions and differing duration of actions

No combination of opioid therapy – regional anesthesia; the sensory block leads to a relative opioid overdosage (respiratory depression)

# MEMORIX SURGERY

## Treatment of chronic pain

### 1. Extending step plan for the treatment of cancer pain
(From Strumpf, M. and Zenz, M.)

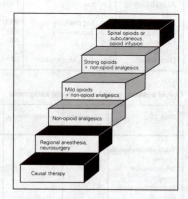

**Aims:**
Freedom from pain
Maintain independence
Increase in activity
Acceptable side effects

The individual dosage regulation attempts to provide continuous freedom from pain

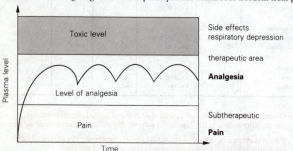

# TREATMENT OF PAIN

**Rules for use of medication in treatment of cancer pain**
- Give medication on a regular basis
  (duration of action = without intervals)
- Assess optimum dosage in steps (requires about 14 days)
- Firm, individual dosage
- As a rule, oral medication
- Exact directions
- Regular check on the effects and side effects
- Anticipate side effects

**Opioid treatment**
**Necessary accompanying medication**

1. Constipation prophylaxis (always)
   e.g. lactulose 2 t.d.s.
2. Antiemetics (intermittent)
   e.g. droperidol

**Equivalent dosages for morphine**

| Application | Relative potency | e.g. mg |
|---|---|---|
| By mouth | 0.33 | 30 |
| i.v./i.m./s.c. | 1 | 10 |
| Epidural | 5 | 2 |
| Intrathecal | 100 | 0.1 |
| Intracerebroventricular | 1000 | 0.01 |

**Example of treatment schedule for cancer pain**

| Drug | Time | Time | Time | Time | Time |
|---|---|---|---|---|---|
| ST 30 3 × 1 tab | 7.00 | | 15.00 | | 23.00 |
| Metoclopramide 3 × 20 | 6.30 | | 14.30 | | 22.30 |
| Lactulose 3 × 2 | 8.00 | 13.00 | | 18.00 | |

## 2. Reflex sympathetic dystrophy

Theory of pain originating in reflex sympathetic dystrophy
(From Blumberg, H. (1988))

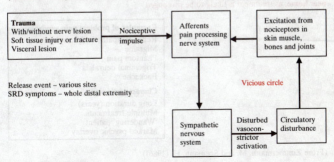

273

# MEMORIX SURGERY

| **Reflex Sympathetic Dystrophy**<br>Autonomic<br>Motor disorders<br>Sensory | Main symptoms:<br>Burning pain<br>Spontaneous pain | As a rule the location of the pain is not restricted to the distribution area of a nerve |

**Treatment:** immediate (success depends on the early institution of treatment)

1. Sympathetic block = causal therapy
2. Ice water compresses
3. Physiotherapy
4. Counter-irritation
5. Balneotherapy

**Sympathetic block (corresponding to site)**
Stellate ganglion – head, upper extremity
Lumbar cord – lower extremity
Intravenous regional anesthesia with
sympatheticolytics (e.g. guanethidine)

| Epidural anesthesia<br>Plexus anesthesia | Additional block of somatosensory afferents |

The verification of the diagnosis should always precede any treatment

### 3. Phantom pain
Similar pain characteristics as in sympathetic reflex dystrophy

| **Immediate treatment**<br><br>Sympathetic block<br>= causal therapy | **Pain prophylaxis**<br>Amputation under regional anesthesia<br>Sympatheticolytics and analgesics<br>for 14 days postoperatively |

4. Patients with problematic pain syndromes require individually organized pain **therapy near home**, as treatment is likely to be prolonged

**Examples of problem pain syndromes**
Reflex sympathetic dystrophy
Migraine
Phantom pain
Trigeminal neuralgia
Backache

**Characteristic signs**
Long duration (years)
Multiple treatments
'Wandering' patient
Marked psychic overlay

(From Zimmermann, M. and Seemann, H. (1986))

# EXPERT OPINIONS AND LEGAL ASPECTS

## Expert opinion

### Assumption

This implies a specific instruction for an expert medico-legal opinion involving directed questioning required, for example, for an accident insurance claim through a trade union, for compensation subsequent to an accident or an occupational disease,

    involving a private accident or insurance claim
    involving pension rights changes or a disablement pension
    involving the certification for the necessity for domiciliary nursing and measures necessary for medical preventive measures and rehabilitation
    in severe incapacitation in persons requiring social security help
    involving compensation under Government compensation
    requiring notification of an infectious disease to avoid further spread
    requiring the discharge of the doctor's duty of secrecy
    the adviser to be expert, objective, independent and experienced, and must, on the basis of his or her ability, be in a position to supply a commissioned opinion

### Example of an expert opinion lay-out

Personal name and address
Date of examination, date of report
Name, address, previous and present occupation of the claimant
Records, references and date of the incident
Person(s) requiring the opinion, and date of request
Type of requested opinion, with listing of special questions
Basis of certification, e.g. medical notes, X-ray films
Diagnosis
Circumstances of the incident, previous history, treatment
Present complaint of the subject
Results of the examination: general and local findings, with requisite measurements
Further specific examination findings (X-rays, laboratory reports, ECG, pulmonary function tests)
A preliminary short critical objective opinion based on a summary of the essential physical and accessory findings
The replies to special questions

# MEMORIX SURGERY

## Legal aspects of surgical practice

### Surgeon–physician–patient relationship
- Consensual – no need to enter into the relationship; however, once it begins, it is difficult to terminate
- Unless patient voluntarily withdraws from the relationship, termination is typically effected after care has been provided and following adequate written notification

### Medical malpractice claims
**Elements**
- Standard of care established; based on professional norms
- Breach of the standard of care in treating a patient
- Injury resulting from the breach
- Patient suffers loss or damage

### Standard of care defined
- National standard in most jurisdictions
- Surgeons are obliged to possess and apply the knowledge and use the skill and care of the reasonable surgeon practicing under the same or similar circumstances

### Typical claims
- Negligent diagnosis or failure to diagnose
- Negligent care and treatment
- Negligent follow-up care
- Negligent failure to refer in time

### Defenses
- Negligence on the part of the patient; may reduce damage award or possibly block any patient recovery
- Statute of limitations has expired
- Surgeon has complied with applicable standard of care
- Other immunities from liability, such as Good Samaritan statute
- Excellent surgeon–patient communication is viewed as one of the most effective risk management techniques and helps avoid many claims

### Consent and informed consent
**From whom**
- Informed consent is to be obtained from the patient, or where necessary, the patient's legal representative (e.g. parent, health-care surrogate, legal guardian)
- Consent is necessary to avoid a claim of battery for unauthorized touching
- Informed consent is necessary to ensure that a patient's consent is knowingly given based on adequate information disclosure

### How obtained
- Surgeon must communicate with patient in a thorough and complete fashion and document the communication in the medical record
- Patient should be offered the opportunity to ask questions and to evidence understanding
- A written informed consent document should be signed by the patient to memorialize the underlying exchange of information

## EXPERT OPINIONS AND LEGAL ASPECTS

**Information disclosure**
- Surgeon should disclose the nature of the proposed procedure, material risks of the procedure, reasonably expected benefits of the procedure, and available alternatives
- In most states, disclosure of information should be consistent with standards of the profession, i.e. what the reasonable practicing surgeon would disclose under the same or similar circumstances
- In almost one-half of the states, disclosure is based on what the reasonable patient would deem to be significant in deciding whether or not to go forward with a particular procedure; the peer or professional-based standard does not control
- Some states have legislation specifically indicating the type of information that must be disclosed

**Documentation and the Medical Record**
**Content of Medical Record**
- Detailed, legible entries signed by the attending surgeon
- Note date and time entry made
- Use standard symbols and abbreviations; avoid unusual abbreviations
- Do not tamper with or make erasures in medical records; corrections should be made with a single line through the incorrect entry together with date and time of cancellation and initials of the person making the modification
- Medical record information should be complete and should also include the content of telephone calls and relevant instructions given to patients

**Ownership of Medical Record**
- Hard copy of medical record belongs to surgeon
- Patient is entitled to review and inspect contents of medical record and to receive photocopy of medical record

# References

Berlit, P. (1991) *Memorix Spezial Neurologie*, VCH, Weinheim.

Berlit, P. (1992) *Neurologie in der Praxis*, VCH, Weinheim.

Bettex, M., Kuffer, E. and Schärli, A.F. (1975) *Wesentliches über Kinderchirurgie*, Huber, Berne.

Bismuth, H. (1988) Surgical anatomy and anatomic surgery of the liver, in *Surgery of the Liver and Biliary Tract* (ed. L.H. Blumgart), Livingstone, London.

Blumberg, H. (1988) Zur Entstehung und Therapie des Schmerzsyndroms bei der sympathischen Reflexdystrophie. *Der Schmerz*, **2**, 125–43.

Braunwald, E. *et al.* (1992) *Heart Diseases*, 4th edn, W.B. Saunders, Philadelphia.

Camp, D. (1931) *Am. J. Roentgenol. Radium Ther.*, **XXVI**(6).

Claudi, B.F. and Oedekoven, G. (1991) Biologische Osteosynthesen. *Chirurgie*, **62**, 367.

Criteria Committee, New York Heart Association (1964) *Diseases of the Heart and Blood Vessels, Nomenclature and Criteria for Diagnosis*, 6th edn, Little Brown, Boston, p. 114.

CUICC (1987) *TNM Classification of Malignant Tumors*, 4th edn, UICC, Geneva.

Dembrowski, U. (1959) Akute arterielle Gefassverschlüsse, in *Angiologie* (ed. M. Ratschow), Thieme, Stuttgart.

Dittler, H.J. and Siewert, J.R. (1990) Erkr. D. Brustdruse, in *Diagnose und Differentialdiagnose in der Chirurgie*, Bd. 2 (eds R. Häring and H. Zilch), VCH, Weinheim.

Dörrler, J. and Hoffmann, G. (1989) Das infrarenale Aortenaneurysma. *Dt. Ärzteblatt*, **86**(19), 1031–6.

Esser, G. and Altmeier, G. (1990) Operatives Vorgehen bei unbekannter Blutungsquelle, in *Gastrointestinale Blutung* (ed. R. Häring), Blackwell Ueberr., Wiss., Berlin.

Editorial (1994) *Blood*, **84**(5), 1361–92.

Empfehlungen der Dt. Ges. F. Pneumologie und Tuberkulose (1987) *Dt. Ärzteblatt*, **84**, A2380.

Emzinger, F. and Weiss, S. (1988) *Soft Tissue Tumors*, 2nd edn, Mosby, St Louis.

Feifel, G. and Gaitrasch, A. (1983) Peritonitis und Infektabwehr. *Chirurgie*, **54**, 298.

Forrest, J.A.H. (1974) Endoscopy in gastrointestinal bleeding. *Lancet*, **ii**, 394.

Freyee, K. and Lammers, W. (1985) *Radiologisches Wörterbuch*, de Gruyter, Berlin and New York.

Froweuin, R.A. *et al.* (1985) Probleme des Hirntodes. *Verh. Dtsch Ges. Neurol. Band.*, **3**, 543–53; Springer, Berlin.

Ghahremani, G.G. and Meyers, M.A. (1975) Internal abdominal hernias, in *Current Problems in Radiology*, vol. V, no. 6 (eds D.H. Baker *et al.*), Year Book Medical Publishers, Chicago.

# REFERENCES

Glintz, W. (1991) Operat. Mögl. Bei der Kniearthroskopie, in Diagn. Und op. Arthroskopie aller Gelenke (eds H. Hempfling and C. Burri), Huber, Berne.

Glinz, W. (1985) Pleuro-pulmonale Verletzungen. *Chirurgie*, **56**, 129.

Grashey, R. and Birkner, R. (1964) *Atlas typischer Röntgenbilder*, Urban and Schwarzenberg, Munchen, Berlin.

Hamann, H. and Volnar, J.F. (1989) Chron. art. Verschlusskrankheit der supraaortalen Äste. *Chirurgie*, **60**, 330–59.

Häring, R. (1990) Erkrankungen der Speiseröhre, in *Diagnose und Differentialdiagnose in der Chirurgie*, vol. 2 (eds R. Häring and H. Zilch), VCH, Weinheim.

Häring, R. and Hirner, A. (1987) Chirurg. Eingriffe beim Pfortaderhochdruck, in *Gefässchirurgie* (eds G. Heberer and R. Van Dongen), Springer, Heidelberg.

Häring, R. and Zilch, H. (1986) *Chirurgie*, De Gruyter, Berlin.

Häring, R. and Zilch, H. (1990) *Diagnose und Differentialdiagnose in der Chirurgie*, vol. 2, VCH, Weinheim.

Hennerici, M. and Neuerberg-Heuser, D. (1988) *Gefassdiagnostik mit Ultraschall*. Thieme, Stuttgart.

Holz, U. and Gieselhart, H. (1992) Becken, Hüftgelenk und Oberschenkel, in *Diagnose und Differentialdiagnose in der Chirurgie* (eds R. Häring and H. Zilch), VCH, Weinheim.

Hunt, W.E. and Hess, R.M. (1968) Surgical risk is related to time of intervention in the repair of intracranial aneurysm. *J. Neurosurg.*, **28**, 14.

Jacoby, G.A. and Swartz, M.N. (1973) Fever of undetermined origin. *N. Engl. J. Med.*, **289**, 1407.

Jennett, B. and Bond, M. (1975) Assessment of outcome after severe brain damage. *Lancet*, p 480.

Jungi, W.F. and Osterwalder, B. (1990) Vorgehen bei Metastasen mit unbekanntem Primärtumor. *Schweiz. Med. Wochenschr.*, **120**, 1273–9.

Kaltenbach, M. and Roskamm, H. (eds) (1980) *Vom Belastungs-EKG zur Koronarangiografie*, Springer, Heidelberg

Konietzko, N. *et al.* (1983) Empfehlungen der Deutschen Gesellschaft für Pneumologie und Tuberkulose. *Prax. Klin. Pneumol.*, **37**, 1199–201.

Loddenkemper *et al.* (1982) Diagnost. Vorgehen beim Pleuraerguss. *Prax. Pneumol.*, **36**, 447.

Lucking, C.H. (1976) Klinische Stadien des Schädel-Hirn-Traumas. *Intensivbehandlung*, **1**, 26.

MacLennan, J.D. (1962) The histotoxic clostridial infections of man. *Bacteriol. Rev.*, **26**, 177.

Martin, M. and Fiebach, B.J.O. (1988) *Die Kurzzeitlyse mit ultrhoher Streptokinase-Dosierung zur Behandlung periph. Arterien.-u. Venenverschlüsse*. Huber, Berne.

Morgan, A.G. and Clamp, S.E. OMGE International upper gastrointestinal bleeding surgery, 1978–1986. *Scand. J. Gastroenterol. (Suppl.)*, **23**, 51.

Müller, M.E. *et al. Manual der Osteosynthese*, 2nd edn, Springer, Heidelberg.

Müller, M.E., Allgöwer, M., Schneider, R. and Willenegger, H. (1992) *Manual der Osteosynthese*, 3rd edn, Springer, Heidelberg and New York.

Muller, R.F., Figley, M.M., Rogoff, S.M. and DeWeese, J.A. Arteries of the abdomen, pelvis and lower extremity. Kodak Publication No. M 4-2. Eastman Kodak Company.

Müller, W. (1982) *Das Knie*, Springer, Heidelberg.

Mumenthaler, M. (1980) *Der Schulter-Arm-Schmerz*, Huber, Berne.

Oppel, F. and Conzen, M. (1990) Neurochirurg. Ekrankungen, in *Diagnose und Differentialdiagnose in der Chirurgie* (eds R. Häring and H. Zilch), VCH, Weinheim.

Rothmund, M. (1990) Endokrine Chirurgie, in *Diagnose und Differentialdiagnose in der Chirurgie* (eds R. Häring and H. Zilch), VCH, Weinheim.

Ruedi, T.H. and Allgöwer, M. (1975) Richtlinien der schweizerischen AO für die Nachbehandlung operativ versorgter Frakturen.

Sarles, H., Gry, K. and Singer, M.V. (1985) *Excerpta Medica*, Elsevier, Amsterdam.

Schwilden, E.D. (1990) Erkrankungen des Venensystems, in *Diagnose und Differentialdiagnose in der Chirurgie* (eds R. Häring and H. Zilch), VCH, Weinheim.

Siewert, R. *et al.* (1979) Stadienerfassung des M. Hodgkin durch Laparotomie. *Chirurgie*, **50**, 478.

Strumpf, M. and Zenz, M. Stufenschema, Btm VV, in *Lehrbuch der Schmerztherapie* (eds M. Zenz and I. Jurna), Wissenschaftliche Verlagsgesellschaft, Stuttgart.

Teasdale, G. and Jennett, B. (1976) Assessment of coma and impaired consciousness. *Acta Neurochir. (Wien)*, **34**, 45.

Thurn, P. and Bücheler, E. (1982) *Einf. In der Röntgendiagnostik*, Thieme, Stuttgart.

Tscherne, E. *et al.* (1987) Schweregrad und Prioritaten bei Mehrfachverletzen. *Chirurgie*, **58**, 631.

Tscherne, H. *et al.* (1988) *Der schwerverletzte Patients – Prioritäten und Management*, Hefte zur Unfallheilk, 200.

Tung, L.C. and Häring, R. (1990) in *Diagnose und Differentialdiagnose in der Chirurgie*, vol. 2 (eds R. Häring and H. Zilch), VCH, Weinheim.

Van Laer, L. (1986) *Frakturen und Luxationen im Wachstumsalter*, Thieme, Stuttgart.

Volmar, J. (1982) *Rekonstruktive Chirurgie der Arterien*, 3rd edn, Thieme, Stuttgart.

Wegener, O.H. (1981) *Computertomographie*, Schering AG.

Zenz, M. (1984) Therapie mit Opiaten, in *Der Schmerz – Konzepte und ärztliches Handeln* (eds H.O. Handwerker and M. Zimmermann), Springer, Berlin, Heidelberg and New York.

Zimmermann, M. and Seemann, H. (1986) Schmerzforschung und schmerztherapeutische Versorgung in der BRD: Defizite und Zukunftsperspektiven,

# REFERENCES

in *Schmerz – Eine interdisziplinäre Herausforderung* (ed. A. Doenick), Springer, Berlin, Heidelberg and New York.

Zuhlke, H. and Hals (1990) in *Diagnose und Differentialdiagnose in der Chirurgie* (eds R. Häring and H. Zilch), VCH, Weinheim.

Zuhlke, H.V. *et al.* (1990) Embol. Gefassverschlüsse im Bereich der Extremitätenarterien. *Akt. Chir.*, **25**, 45–50.

# INDEX

## Index

Abdomen 23, 30
  arteries 175
  X-rays 23, 30
    colonic ileus 30
    upper ileal ileus 30
    lower ileal ileus 30
Abdominal aorta aneurysm 235
Abdominoperineal rectum resection 158
Abscess 177
  perianal 178
  retroperitoneal 177
Acetylsalicylic acid 271
Achalasia 30
Adamantinoma 206
Adductor slit 234
Adhesiolysis 69
Adhesion ileus 67
Adiposity, risk factor 161
Adrenal cortex 225
Adrenogenital syndrome 223
AIDS 91
Aitken classification 189
Acanthocytes 174
Acromegaly 225
Acromioclavicular joint 22
  injury 22
Acoustic neuroma 255
Acute extremity artery ischemia 236
Acute peripheral artery obstruction 235
  diagnosis 236
  etiology 235
  symptoms 235
  treatment 236
Acute abdomen 142
  definition 142
  diagnosis 143
  extra-abdominal differential diagnosis 143
  symptoms 142
  site differential diagnosis 144
Algodystrophy 193
Alcoholic hallucinations 248
Ampulla of Vater carcinoma 162
  TNM classification 162
Amputations 212
Anal carcinoma 178
  TNM classification 178
Anal polyps 179
Anemia 18
  diagnosis 18
  etiology 18
  macrocytic 18
  microcytic 18
  normocytic 18
  treatment 18
  counseling premedication
Anastomosis, mammarocoronary 102
Anastomotic carcinoma 154
Aneurysm, arterial 227f
  diagnosis 228
  false 227
  classification 227
  spurious 227
  treatment 228
  dissecting 236
  differential diagnosis 236
Angioblastoma (Lindau) 255
Angiography 37
  preparation 37
Angioma 255
Ankle arterial pressure 236
Ann Arbor classification 244
Annular pancreas 62
Anterior rectal resection 158
Anterior tibial syndrome 207
Antifibrinolytics 20
Anticoagulent medication, upper gastrointestinal bleeding 54
Anticoagulation 240
  indications 240
  contraindications 240
Artificial anus 159f
  complications 160
  sigmoid 158
AO classification of fractures 184
AO principle 180
Aortic dissection 235
Aortic isthmus stenosis 97, 100
  operative technique 100
  symptoms 100
Aortic stenosis 97
Apnea 246
Appendicectomy 69
Apprehension test 195
Apud system 224
Apudoma 268
  tumor marker 268
Arnold–Chiari deformity 256
Arterial block 231
Arterial emboli 235
  differential diagnosis 236
Arterial thrombosis 235
  differential diagnosis 236
Arterial vascular system 226
  auscultation 226
Arteries
  abdomen 175
  leg 233
  pelvis 232
Arterioportal fistula 167
Arthritis 31
  differential diagnosis 31
  X-rays 31
Ascaris 54

# INDEX

Ascendodescendostomy 158
Astrocytoma 255
Asystole 49
  resuscitation 49
Atropine 246
Auto-immune disease 54
A–V canal 97
Axial skin graft 209
Azygos vein 25

Babcock vein stripping 243
Baker's cyst 197
Balloon septostomy 99
Bankart's lesion 45, 94
Basal cisterns 254
Basophil granulations 174
Bassi perforators 241
Baxter scheme 58
Berger–Kunert system 75
Bile duct carcinoma
  hepatocellular 165
  intrahepatic 165
  primary 165
Bile duct diseases 161
  operation indications 161
Bilharziasis 167
Biliodigestive anastomosis 162
Billroth-I operation 148
Billroth-II operation 148
Bjork–Shiley flap 105
Blalock–Taussig 99
Bleeding 65, 92, 255
  acute subdural 255
  chronic subdural 255
  ear 92
  epidural 255
  mouth 92
  nose 92
  peranal 65
  subarachnoid 255
Bleeding time (Duke) 19
Blood picture, normal 17
  differential 17
Blood dyscrasia 54
  GI bleeding 54
Blood sedimentation rate 17
Blowout fracture 22, 92
Bones
  fractures 182
  healing time 182
Bone defect 210f
  longitudinal 211
Bone necrosis
  aseptic 204
  Dietrich 204
  Friedrich 204
  Haas 204
  Kienböck 204
  Köhler I 204
  Köhler II 204
  Osgood–Schlatter 204
  Panner 204
  Perthes 204
  Preiser 204
  Scheuermann 204
  Sinding–Larsen–Johannsson 204
  Thiemann 204
Bone nucleus 32
Bone tumors 206f
  operative indications 206
  TNM classification 206
Borrmann classification 151
Bowen's disease 179
Brain arteries 252
Brain death criteria 264
Brain infarct 248
Brain lesions 205
Brain pressure 256
Brain tumors 255
Braun enteroanastomosis 148
Brock 99
Bronchial carcinoma 122, 268
  TNM classification 122
  tumor marker 268
Bronchial tree 117
  lobes 117
  lymph nodes 117
  segments 117
Bronchoscope 120
Bronchoscopy 118
Budd–Chiari syndrome 167
Bulbar syndrome 250f
Bulb, blood supply 150
Buprenorphine 271

Burns 57, 60
Burst abdomen 140
Buschke–Lowenstein tumor 179
Buttonhole deformity 216
Bypass 234, 237
  anatomic 237
  extra-anatomic 237

Calcaneus
  posterior 36
  anterior 36
Callus distraction 211
Callus formation 181
Calor (heat) 84
Capitulate bone 35
Carcinoid 224
Cardiac carcinoma 30
Cardiac insufficiency 60
Cardiopulmonary resuscitation 48
Carlen's tube 123
Caroli's syndrome 166
Carotid stenosis, sonography 230
Carpal tunnel syndrome 195, 261
Catatonia 248
Cauda equina 263
  injury 200
Cerebral aneurysm 253
  common sites 253
  pathogenesis 253
  treatment 253
Cerebral circulation insufficiency 229
  classification 229
  operative indication 229
Cervical rib 195
Cervical spine 257
Cervical vertebra 22
Chassaignac injury 194
Cheyne–Stokes breathing 246
Children's surgery
  adhesion ileus 61
  annular pancreas 62
  bleeding, peranal 65
  congenital lobar emphysema 64
  duodenal atresia 62
  duodenal membrane 62

# INDEX

dyspnea 64
emergency 61ff
foreign-body aspiration 64
hiatus hernia 61
incarcerated inguinal hernia 62
invagination 61
jejunal atresia 62
malrotation 62
meconium ileus 62
necrotizing enterocolitis 63
pylorus stenosis hypertrophic 61
relaxed diaphragm symptoms 64
scrotum, acute 65
stress pneumothorax 64
toxic megacolon 63
tracheal stenosis 64
volvulus 62
Child's classification 56
Cholangiography 161
Cholelithiasis 161
  complications 161
  diagnosis 161
  risk factors 161
  treatment 161
Cholecystectomy 69
Cholesterol 161
Chondropathia of patella 197
Chondrosarcoma 206
Chopart's lines 212
Chordoma 206
Chorion carcinoma 268
Chronic myeloid leukemia 174
Chronic venous insufficiency 242
Cimini shunt 238
Clamp suture 16
Clark classification melanoma 77
*Clostridium* cellulitis 86
*Clostridium* myonecrosis 86
Coccydinia 179
Cockett perforators 241
Codeine 271
Colon, lymph nodes 158

Colorectal carcinoma 157, 268
  frequency 157
  localization 157
  TNM classification 157
  tumor marker 268
Colson flap 219
Coma 250
Compartment syndrome 202, 207
Computed tomography 37
Condylar plate 196
Condylomata acuminata 179
Congenital lobar emphysema 64
Coniotomy 53
Conn's syndrome 223
Continence resection 172
Coronary arteries, nomenclature 101
Coronary heart disease, operative indications 102
Coronary obstruction treatment 101
Corticospongiosa chips 210
  complications 210
  removal sites 210
Coumarin 20
Craniopharyngioma 255
Crohn's disease 155
Cruciate ligament 45
Crutchfield extensor 201, 254
Cryptitis 179
Cushing's syndrome 223
Cystojejunostomy 171
Cytology 267

Daniel's classification 87
Death, time of 264
DeBakey's classification 227
Decubitus ulcer predilection sites 87
Deep pelvic and femoral venous thrombosis 239f
Defect covering 209
Defects, bones 210, 211

Demer's catheter 238
Dens (axis) 22
Dens screw 259
Dermatitis 159
Dermoid 255
Dermoid cyst 179
Descendorectostomy 158
Dextropropoxyphen 271
Diagnosis security 266
Diaphragm 139
  classification 137
  deficiency 139
  hernia 64, 137
  predilection for defects 139
  treatment 137
Diclofenac 271
Differential diagnosis of edema 242
Dihydrocodeine 271
Dilated pupils 251
Disc hernia 262
  lateral 262
  medial 262
  mediolateral 262
  operation indications 262
Disc prolapse 263
Dissecting aneurysm 236
  differential diagnosis 236
Diverticuli 135, 156
  abstraction of 156
  cervical 135
  epiphrenal 135
Diverticulitis 172
  complications 172
  treatment 172
Diverticulosis 172
Dodd grouping 241
Dolor (pain) 84
Donor blood 68
Doppler sonography 230, 239, 242
  carotid stenosis 230
  inguinal 239
  varicose veins 242
  venous 239
Dor's operation 103
Dorsal fixation 259
Dragstedt mechanism 148
Drainage operations 171

# INDEX

Ductus arteriosus Botalli 97
Ductus Botalli, open 100
Duke's classification 157
Dumping syndrome 154
   early dumping 154
   late dumping 154
Dual head prosthesis 196
Duodenal atresia 62
Duodenal membrane 62
Duodenal stump 154
   remaining antral mucosa 154
Duodenal ulcer 149
Dupuytren's contracture 217
Duval's operation 171
Dynamic hip screw 196
Dyspepsia 161
Dysphagia, diagnosis 135

Ear canals 22
   external 22
   internal 22
Ebstein anomaly 97
Echinococcus 54
Echymoses 19
Eisenmenger complex 98
Edema 242
Elbow 23
   coronoid process 23
   radial head
   X-rays
Elbow dislocation 194
Electromechanical dissociation, resusitation 49
Electromyography 261
Elliptocytosis 174
Emergencies, spinal 258
   symptoms 258
   treatment 259
Emergency sonography 42
Encephalitis 248
Encephalopathy, hepatic 56
Enchondroma 206
Endosonography 42
Ependymoma 255
Epicondylitis 195
Epididymitis 65
Epidural hematoma 248

Epiphyses 32
   epiphyseal closure 32
Epiphysis fracture 189
Epsilon-aminocaproic acid 20
ERCP 161
Ergotism 235
Esophageal carcinoma 30
Esophageal spasm 30
Esophageal varicose bleeding 56
Esophagitis 137
   classification 137
   complications 137
   stenosis 30
Esophagus 30, 135f, 138
   anatomy 135
   atresia 136
   carcinoma 138
      TNM classification 138
      treatment 138
   diagnosis 136
Ewing's sarcoma 206
Extrahepatic bile duct, carcinoma 162
   TNM classification 162
Extrapyramidal lesions 205

Facial fractures 92
Facial skull 22
Fallot's tetrology 97, 99
   treatment 99
Fascial flaps 75
Fascial splitting 208
Femoral fractures 194
Femoral neck fractures 196
Femoral prostheses 196
Fever of unknown origin 89
   collagen diseases 89
   local infection 84
   neoplasia 84
   systemic infection 84
Fibrin stabilization test 19
Fibrosarcoma 206
Finger-floor test 5
Fissure 179
Fistula 160, 178
   artificial anus 160

   perianal 178
Flexion-distraction trauma 200
Flexure resection 158
Fluid requirement, intraoperative 68
Fontaine staging 231
Foramen of Luschke 256
Foramen of Magendie 256
Foramen magnum 22
Forrest's classification 55
Fracture healing, complications 181
Fracture treatment, conservative 191
Fractures 180, 202
   complications 202
   diagnosis 180
   osteosynthesis 202
   postoperative further treatment 202
   treatment methods 180
      conservative 180
      operative 180
Free fibula transfer 211
Free skin grafting 209
Foreign-body aspiration 64

Galactorrhea 225
Ganglion, knee 197
Garden's classification 196
Gardner's syndrome 159
Gas-forming wound infection 86
Gastrinoma 154, 224
Gastroenteroanastomosis 148
Gastrografin 37
Gastrointestinal bleeding 54f
   lower 54
      diagnosis 54
      differential diagnosis 54
   upper 54f
      causes 54
      esophageal varices 55
      ulcer 54
Gastrojejunostomy 148
Gastroschisis 135
Genital organs, injury 196

# INDEX

Germ cell tumor marker 268
Glasgow coma scale 247
Glasgow outcome scale 247
Glioblastoma multiforme 255
Glucagonoma 224
Goodpasture's syndrome 128
Grading 266
Grand mal 248
Granulation tissue 83
Granuloma venereum 179
Granulomatous colitis 159

Habitual shoulder dislocation 194
Hach's classification 241
Hamate bone 35
Hand 23, 214ff
  anesthesia 214
  chronic diseases 217
  infections 218
  navicular quartet 23
  tendons 216
  tendon injuries 216
  wound closure 219
  X-rays 23
Hand bones 35
  access 35
Hand joints 35, 211
  anatomy 211
  joint angle 35
Hartmann's operation 172
Hashimoto's thyroiditis 44
Heart defects 97ff
  acyanotic group 97
  congenital 97ff
    acyanotic group with shunt 98
    'blue' 99
    cyanotic group with shunt (right–left) 99
    overview 97
    'white' 98
Heart–lung machine 113
Heart transplantation indications 105
Heart trauma 114
  blunt 114

sharp 114
  treatment 114
Heart tumors 112
  diagnosis 112
  frequency 112
  operative methods 112
  symptoms 112
Heart valves, auscultation 105
Heart valve defects 101, 104
  acquired 104
    aortic valve 104
    mitral valve 104
    tricuspid valve 104
  diagnosis 100
  internal 139
  treatment 104
Heinz bodies 174
Hemangioma 206
Hemangiopericytoma 206
Hematemesis, differential diagnosis 128
Hematoma, retroperitoneal 177, 196
Hemicolectomy 158
  left 158
  right 158
Hemobilia, causes 54
Hemoptysis 128
  diagnosis 128
  differential diagnosis 128
Hemorrhoids 179
Hemostiologic diagnosis 19
  basic diagnosis 19
  laboratory diagnosis 19
Heparin 20
Hernia 140f
  anatomy 141
  definition 140
  differential diagnosis 140
  internal 141
Hernia, operations 69
Hiatus hernia 61
Hill-Sachs-Dent 194
Hip, X-rays 24
  ala 24
  Lauenstein 24
  obturator view 24

Hip joint dislocation 45
Hydatid torsion 65
Hydatidiform mole 268
Hydrocephalus 255
  communicating 256
  occlusive 256
Hypercortisonism 225
Hypergastrinemia, diagnosis 225
Hyperlipidemia 169
Hyperparathyroidism 154, 167, 169, 222
  causes 222
  diagnosis 222
  risk factors 161
  symptoms 222
  treatment 222
Hyperpigmentation 225
Hypertension, portal 167
  collateral circulation 167
Hyperthyroidism 220, 225
  operation preparation 220
Hypocalcemia 222
  hyperparathyroidism 222
Hypophyseal tumors 225, 255

Ibuprofen 271
Ileal anastomosis 156
Ileocecal resection, Crohn 161
  risk factors 161
Ileostomy 159
Ileostomy fistula 159
Ileo-transverseostomy 158
Ileum 155f
  anastomosis 156
  laterolateral 156
  operations on 156
  resection 156
  resorption 155
    albumin, fat 155
    disaccharides
    electrolytes 155
    fat-soluble vitamins 155
    monosaccharides 155
    water-soluble vitmines 155
  terminolateral 156

# INDEX

terminoterminal 156
tumors 155
Ileus 146
  causes 147
  definition 146
  diagnosis 146
  operations 146
  treatment 146
Immunothrombocytopenic purpura 174
Impingement syndrome 195
Incarcerated inguinal hernia 62
Incontinence resection 172
Infected vascular gangrene 86
Inflammation, chronic 161
Inflammation, signs 84
Infratentorial space 246
Injection 9ff
  intra-articular 9
Injection bronchoscope 120
Insertion tendonopathy knee 197
*In situ* bypass 234
Insulinoma 224
Intraluminal stents 237
Invagination 61
IRINS (irreversible ischemic neurological symptoms) 229

Jaundice 166
  classification 166
  diagnosis 166
  differential diagnosis 166
  intrahepatic 166
  posthepatic 166
Jejunal atresia 62
Johnson classification 148
Joint bodies, free 31
Joint punctures 10f
  elbow 10
  hand 10
  hip 11
  knee 11
  shoulder 10

Kanavels sign 218

Karnovsky index 265
Kiel classification 245
Kirchmaer suture 216
Knee 24, 197f
  anatomy 198
  arthroscopy 198
  free joint bodies 197
  trauma 197
  tunnel view (Frick) 24
Kocher's collar-stud suture 73
Korsakow's syndrome 248

Labyrinth 22
Labyrinth deficit 205
Lachmann test 195
Langer's skin ines 71
Laparoscopic appendicectomy 70
Laparoscopic cholecystectomy 70
Laparoscopic surgery 69
Lauren classification 151
Legal aspects of surgical treatment 276
Leio-myosarcoma 206
Leukemia 54
  gastrointestinal bleeding, upper 54
Leukemic reticuloendotheliosis 174
Levomethadone 271
Life quality 267
Linton's line 241
Linton's shunt 168
Lipoma 206
Liposarcoma 206
Lisfranc line 212
Littre–Richter hernia 140
Liver 163f
  anatomy 163
  standard resections 164
  vascular supply 163
    anatomical variations 163
Liver cell carcinoma tumor marker 268
Liver cirrhosis 166f
Liver tumors 165
Local recurrences 266
Local/regional flap plasty 209
Longmire–Gutgemann reconstruction 153
Lower abdominal incision for extraperitoneal approach 73
Lower midline lapartomy incision with navel extension 73
Lumbar vertebrae 26
Lungs 119f, 124
  lobes 119
  parenchyma fistula 124
  segments 119
  staging 120
  tumor diagnosis 120
Lung embolus 131f
  diagnosis 131
  etiology 131
  protective operation 132
  staging 132
  symptoms 131
Lung funciton 116
  additional investigations 116
  basic diagnosis 116
Lung surgery procedures 123
Lung tumors, WHO classification 121
Lymphangioma 206
Lymph node involvement 261
Lymphoma in neck area
  diagnosis 93
  surgical anatomy 94

Macrohematuria 21
Magnetic resonance tomography 39ff
  basis 39
  contraindications 40
  indications 40
  spinal cord 41
Maisonneuve fracture 199
Malgaigne's furrow 194
Malignant melanoma 78
  diagnosis 78
  treatment 78
Mallory–Weiss syndrome 54
Malrotation 62

# INDEX

Marseille classification 169
Mass movement 250
Massive bleeding 248
Mastoid process 22
Mathes–Nahai classification 76
Maxillary clamping 92
Maxillary fracture 92
May perforans 241
Maydl hernia 140
Meconium ileus 62
Median sternotomy 73
Mediastinal tumors 125f
  classification 125
  diagnosis 126
  sites, diagnosis 126
Mediastinoscopy 120
Mediastinum, anatomy 126
Medullary thyroid carcinoma 225, 268
  tumor marker 268
Medulloblastoma 255
Melanoma 77
  Clark classification 77
Meningioma 255
Meningitis 248
Meniscus injury 45
Mesenteric tumor, malassimilation syndrome in 155
Metabolic disorders 246
Metal splint removal 198
Metamizol 271
Metastases 255, 269
  brain 255
  spinal cord 255
  unknown primary tumor 269
Microhematuria 21
Microspherocytes 174
Microvascular flap plasty 209
Midbrain syndrome 250f
Miles' classification 179
Millesi classification 260
Mirizzi's syndrome 166
Monocular hematoma 92
Morphine 271, 273
  equivalent dosages 273
Multiple myeloma, tumor marker 268

Myelofibrosis 174
Myocutaneous flap 75
Myxoma 206

Nalbuphin 271
Naloxone 271
Nasal bone, fracture 92
Natural death 277
Necrosis, artificial anus 160
Necrosing enterocolitis 63
Nerve compression syndrome, peripheral 261
  diagnosis 261
  symptoms 261
  treatment 261
Nerve conduction velocity 261
Neuner's rule 52
Neurinoma 206, 250
Neuroblastoma 268
Neurogenic sarcoma 201
Neuroleptanalgesia 66
Neutral-zero method 2
Non-Hodgkin lymphoma 245
Non-opioids 270
NYHA classification 109

Oligodendroglioma 255
Open bite 92
Opiates 246
Opioids 270
Opioid treatment 273
Orbital hematoma 92
Ormond's disease 177
Osgood–Schlatter's disease 197
Ossification 32
Osteoblastoma 206
Osteochondroma 206
Osteoid osteoma 206
Osteoma 206
Osteosarcoma 206
Osteosynthesis 192
Ovarian carcinoma 268
Ovulation inhibitors 239

Pacchioni granules 256
Paget's disease 179
Pancoast tumor 195

Pancreas 169
Pancreas, carcinoma tumor marker 268
Pancreas, operations 171
Pancreas, tumors 170
  endocrine 224
  TNM classification 170
  WHO classification 170
Pancreatitis 155, 169
  acute 169
  chronic 169
  Malassimilation syndrome 155
Papanicolaou classification 267
Papillary stenosis 166
Papillitis 179
Paracetamol 271
Paraganglioma 225
Paralysis, abdominal examination 30
Pararectal incision 73
Parastomal hernia 159
Parathormone 222
  hyperparathyroidism 222
Pareses 263
Parkinson gait 205
Parkinson's disease 133
  dysphagia 135
Parona phlegmone 218
Paronychia 218
Patella, X-rays 24
Patty's operation 134
Pelvic floor, hernia 139
Pelvic fractures 196
Pelvis 24
  arteries 232
Percutaneous endoscopic gastrostomy 153
Percutaneous transluminal coronary angioplasty 102
Perforating veins 241
Perforation, artificial anus, complication 160
Perianal thrombosis 179
Perianal hematoma 179
Pericardial effusion, symptoms 115
Pericardial puncture technique 115

# INDEX

Perineal closure 158
Peristomal hernia 160
Peritonitis 145
 definition 145
 symptoms 145
 treatment 145
Perthes test 242
Pes anserinus 234
Petechiae 19
Pethidine 271
Petit's hernia 140
Pfannenstiel incision 73
Phaechromocytoma 224
Phantom pain 274
 prophylaxis 270
Phlebography 37
Phlegmasia dolens 230f
 diagnosis 236
Pilonidal sinus 179
Pineal tumors 255
Piritramid 271
Pituitary tumors 223, 255
Plaster bandaging 191
Platform epithelium tumor marker 268
Pleural effusion 44, 127
 diagnosis 127
Plexus lesion 260
 diagnosis 260
 treatment 260
Polyposis 159
Polytrauma 50ff
 general 50f
 multiple 52
Popliteal artery 233
Popliteal bursitis 197
Positioning 47
Posterior tibial syndrome 207
Postoperative fever 88
Post-splenectomy sepsis 174
Prechtel's classification 133
Prepatellar bursitis 197
Principle of biological osteosynthesis 180, 192
Principles of the AO technique 192
PRIND (prolonged ischemic neurological defect 229
Proctalgia 179
Proctitis 179
Proctocolectomy 155, 173
 malabsorption syndrome 155
Procto-colitis ulcerosa 179
Proctology 178
Prolapse 140
 anus, rectum 179
Pronator teres syndrome 261
Prostatic carcinoma, tumor marker 268
Prosthesis care 212
Protamine 20
Proxen 271
Pseudoarthrosis 181, 202
 atrophic 181
 defect 181
 hypertrophic 181
 oligotrophic 181
Pseudocysts 169
Puestow's operation 171
Pugh's classification 56
Pulvertaft's suture 216
Pupil width 251
Purpura 19
Pyloric stenosis, hypertrophic 61
Pyodermia fistulans 179

Quadriceps tendon lesions 45

Radius, fracture 193
 osteosynthesis 193
 reduction 193
Rashkind 99
Ratschow's position 231
Rectosigmoid resection 158
Recurrent carcinoma 160
Regional anesthesia 66, 270
Re-implantation 213
 indication 213
 procedure 213
Resuscitation 48
 diagnosis 48
 emergency 48
 immediate measures 48
Retraction, in artificial anus 160
Retroperitoneal fibrosis 177
Retroperitoneal vascular injury 196
Rheumatism, hand 217
Rhythm disorders 107f
 bradycardia 107
 medication treatment 107
 pacemaker 107
 operative approach 107
 tachycardia 108
 anti-arrhythmic surgery 108
Rib border incision 73
Riedel goitre 44
Rotation endarteriectomy 237
Rotation/transposition flap 209
Rotator cuff 195
Roux's sling 148
Rubor (redness) 84
Rumpel–Leede test 19

Sacral vertebrae 257
Scalenus deficiency 195
Scaphoid bone 35
Scar 57
 hypertrophy 57
Scar severity 57
Schanz cravat 259
Schatzki ring, dysphagia 135
Scintography 37
Segmental innervation 257
Seiler's classification 87
Sellick's maneuver 67
Seminoma 268
Sensory disorders 263
Septum resection after Blalock–Hanlon 99
Shober's sign 5
Shock 46
 classification 46
 definition 46
 index 46
 symptoms 46

# INDEX

Shoulder 22f
  Bankart lesion 23
  Hill-Sachs-Delle 23
  X-rays 23
    transthoracic 23
    Y-view 23
Shoulder arm pain 190
Shoulder dislocation 45
Sickle-cell anemia 174
Siewert-Peiper reconstruction 153
Sigma resection 158
Sigmoidorectostomy 158
Sigmoidostomy 159
Sinding-Larsen-Johannsson syndrome 197
Skin carcinoma, TNM classification 77
Skin graft flap 75
  classification 75
Soleus curve 234
Somatosensitive evoked potential (SEP) 261
Somatostatinoma 224
Somnolence 250
Sonography 42ff
  adrenals 44
  breast 44
  emergency 42
  indications 42
  endosonography 42
  gallbladder 43
  great abdominal vessels 44
  hip 45
  kidneys 44
  knee 45
  ligaments 45
  liver 43
  muscles 45
  soft tissues 45
  spleen 43
  thorax 44
  thyroid 44
Space-occupying lesions, intracerebral 255
Sparing operations 132
Spherocytosis 174
Spinal canal, narrowing 201
Spinal cord tumors 255

Spinal emergencies 258f
  symptoms 258
  treatment 259
Splenectomy 174
Spondylosis 195
Spongiosa screw 196
Spongiosa transplant 210
  complications 210
  taking sites 210
Staging operation 244
Standard operations, colorectal 158
Stanford classification 227
Starr-Edwards flap 105
Stenosis 160
  artificial anus 160
  contralateral 229
Stenver's X-ray view 22
Steppe walk 205
Sternum, X-rays 22
St Jude medical flap 105
Stomach 152, 154
  lymph nodes 152
  operated 154
  vessels 152
Stomach, carcinoma 151, 153, 268
  classification 151
  reconstruction 153
  resections 153
  TNM classification 151
  tumor marker 268
Stomach remnant 154
Stomach ulcer 148
Streptococcal myositis 86
Streptokinase 20
Stretch inhibition 197
  free joint bodies 197
  knee 197
Stump carcinoma 154
Subarachnoid bleeding 248, 254
  classification 254
Subclavian vessels, approach 73
Subdural hematoma 248
Subtotal pancreatectomy 171
Subumbilical transverse incision 73
Sudeck's disease 193
Sunderland classification 260

Supinator syndrome 261
Suprainguinal incision 73
Suture material 13
  absorbable 13
  atraumatic 13
  monofil 13
  non-absorbable 13
  polyfil 13
  pseudomonofil 13
  traumatic 13
Suture technique 14f
  Allgower suture 14
  Donati suture 14
  gastrointestinal suture 15
  intradermal suture 14
  knot suture 14
  mattress suture 14
  principles 14
  sling suture 14
  suture removal
Syme's lines 212
Sympathetic block 274
Sympathetic reflex dystrophy 181, 193, 195, 202, 273
Syndrome of the blind sling 155
Syndrome of Loge de Guyon 261
Synovitis, knee 197
Syringomyelia 195

Target cells 174
Tarsal tunnel syndrome 261
T-cell lymphoma 245
T-drain insertion 162
Temporal lobe fainting 248
Tendopathy/synovitis 217
Tenosynovitis 217
Tensor fasciae latae 75
Teratoma 268
Tetanus 85
  immunization 85
  staging 85
Thalassemia 174
Thallium scintography 97
Thoracic outlet syndrome 261

# INDEX

Thoracic vertebrae 257
Thorax drainage 124
 indications 124
 technique 124
Thorax, injury treatment 130
Thorax, pain diagnosis 129
Thorax, transverse incision 73
Thorax, X-rays 23, 25
 azygos vein lobe 25
 sources of error 23
Thrombasthenia 19
Thrombectomy 240
 contraindications 240
 indications 240
Thrombendarteriectomy 234, 237
 contraindications 240
 indications 240
Thrombocyte function 19
Thrombocytopenia 19
Thrombolysis 240
Thyroid 220
 anatomy 220
 classification 221
 diagnosis 220
 operative indications 220
Thyroid carcinoma 221
 anaplastic 221
 follicular 221
 medullary 221
 papillary 221
Transient ischemic attacks (TIA) 229
Tiffeneau test 116
Tilidine 271
TNM classification, melanoma 77
Tossy classification 195
Total endoprosthesis 196
Toxic hepatitis 166
Toxic megacolon 63
Tracheal stenosis 64
Tracheostomy 53
Tramadol 271
TRAM, transverse rectus abdominis muscle 75
Tranexaminic acid 20
Transport of amputate 213

Transposition of the great vessels 99
 treatment 99
Transposition flap plasty 74
Transverse resection 158
Transversosigmoidostomy 73
Trapping procedure 253
Trauma 83
 blunt 81
 sharp, pointed 83
Traumatic vascular contraction 236
Trendelenburg limp 205
Trendelenburg test 241
Trigeminal neuralgia 274
TRINS (total reversible ischemic neurological symptoms) 229
Truncus arteriosus 99
Tube implantation (Celestin, Haring) 153
Tube stenosis 166
Tuberculosis 169
Tumor (swelling) 84
Tumor marker 268
Tumor therapy 267
TVS de Quervain 217
Tytgatt catheter 162

Ulcer 150
 acute bleeding 150
 perforating 150
Ulcer, surgery 148ff
 elective 148 f
Ulcerative colitis 159, 169, 173
Ulcerative coloproctitis 179
Ulnar syndrome 261
Umbilical hernia 140
 fistula 140
Univentricular heart treatment 99
Upper abdominal transverse incision 73
Upper ankle joint 24
 talus tipping 24
 talus stubbing 24

Urachus fistula 140
Uremia, upper GI bleeding 54
Urinary sediment 21
Urine 21
Urokinase 20

Vagotomy 144, 147
 incomplete 147
 proximal 144
 technique 144
Valvular congenital heart defects 97
Varicose veins 241ff
 treatment, technique 243
Vascular block 234
Vascular closure 234
 surgery, treatment 234
Vascular surgery, technique 237
Vein bypass, aortocoronary 102
Venereal granuloma 179
Venography 37
Venous access 12
Ventricle-paced pacemakers 108
Ventral fusion 259
Ventricular septum defect 98
 frequency 98
 localization 98
Ventriculoatrial shunt 256
Ventriculoperitoneal shunt 256
Vertebrae normal development 34
Vertebral column, angles of movement 5
 MRI of 41
Vipoma 224
Visceral arterial block 176
Volkmann's contracture 207
Volume replacement, intraoperative 68
Volvulus 62, 147
Vomiting in children 61
V–Y-flap 74, 75

Weber fractures 199

# INDEX

WHO classification
  of lung tumors 121
  of esophageal tumors 138
  of pancreatic tumors 170
von Willebrand's disease 19
Wound healing 83
  disorders of 84
Wound infections, gas-forming 86
Wounds
  in burns 57
  management of 83
Wrist bones 35
Wrist
  joint punctures 10

X-ray diagnosis
  routine 22

Y photographs 23
Y–V-plasty 74, 75

Zollinger–Ellison syndrome 154, 225
Z-plasty 74, 75